That Time of Year

The University of Massachusetts Press, 1982

That Time of Year

A CHRONICLE OF LIFE IN A NURSING HOME

Joyce Horner

That Time of Year has been transcribed for
publication with minimal editorial alterations.
Three poems written before the author's illness
have been added; the names of the nursing home
staff and patients, and of their families and
friends, have been changed. Acknowledgment
for permission to reprint material in copyright
is listed on pages 206–7.

Copyright © 1982 by
The University of Massachusetts Press
All rights reserved
Printed in the United States of America
LC 81–23128   ISBN 0–87023–367–X

Summer People

If we could stay
Here always in this meadow
Under this tree,
Here in woodland shallows of fern and bay
And by a silk-sewn sea,
Riders through *mille-fleurs* fields in endless leisure—
Wild rose and berries and the wings
Of small things under the leaves—
In a trance of pleasure;
If we could stay
Waist-deep in grass where Queen Anne's lace is
The height of a child's eye,
We could be
The people in blue-green and flat gold leaf
Safe under the paradise tree.
But the breath comes and goes, even the breath
Of summer, and when the cold
Drives the deer from their hiding places
To seek the apples
Under this tree,
And the hunters crash through the alders to the water
With powerful hands and stern faces,
We shall not be here to see.
We are summer people
Who go home in winter.

Introduction

The biographical facts of Professor Joyce Mary Horner's life (July 13, 1903–March 24, 1980) may be very briefly sketched.* She was born in Lofthouse, Yorkshire, England. She attended both Guiseley School and Leeds Girls' High School; then, after taking her undergraduate degree at St. Hilda's, Oxford, acquired a Master of Arts at Smith College in the United States. In the summers of 1941–1943, she participated in the University of New Hampshire Writers' Conference at Durham. She had taught in Canada, Texas, and at Hood College in Frederick, Maryland, before joining the English faculty at Mount Holyoke College in 1944. At Mount Holyoke in South Hadley, Massachusetts, she remained until her retirement, as a full professor, in 1969. She published two novels, *The Wind and the Rain* and *The Greyhound in the Leash*, and occasionally placed poetry in leading magazines. Her chief interest in teaching, combined with her constant enjoyment of good literature, was in composition—particularly "the structure of the English sentence" in both fine prose and poetry. While at a hospital for tests after her retirement, she suffered a fall, breaking several bones; a semi-invalid as a result of this and her continuing arthritis, she left her home in South Hadley and en-

* I am indebted for information and other aid in my consideration of this text and its author to Elizabeth Green (Professor Emeritus of Mount Holyoke College) and to Ben L. Reid (Professor of English at Mount Holyoke).

tered, on June 18, 1974, a nursing home about fifteen miles away, but still in Massachusetts' Connecticut River Valley.

These are the "facts," but a fuller, richer conception of those aspects in her life that meant most to Joyce Horner can be gathered from the present chronicle of her experience at the nursing home, a chronicle she kept more and more intermittently from March 11, 1975, until June 27, 1977. The journal ends with her anticipating a move to a Boston hospital for a knee operation (which proved impossible).

The most remarkable feature of Joyce Horner's writing here seems to me the indelible impression it leaves of her resilience of spirit. There is, of course, the poignancy of her increasing physical disability in the company of other ailing elderly persons, the poignancy of her growing realization of mortality. But beyond her unflinching recognition of death's approach, what stands out even more during the course of the chronicle is the sure recurrence of Joyce Horner's vital attention to everything perceivable around her.

She brings to all her perceptions in these latter years the strengths of a lively mind long imbued in Classical and English literature and in the Liberal Arts generally. She also retains vivid memories of her childhood, youth, and professional career—including welcome vacations: summers with her mother at Brighton beach in England, more recent ones on the Maine coast with her friends, Cunard liner crossings, trips to Greece, Sicily, Italy, Paris. She treasures, still, occasional visits home (the South Hadley home she had shared with her dearest friend and colleague, Elizabeth), enjoys receiving visitors (Elizabeth and other friends) at the nursing home, values letters from relatives and former students.

Her will to stir the dull roots, to overcome the routine inertias of the nursing home and the fatiguing discomforts of age, is evidenced by her continuing to write, not only her prose chronicle but the poetry in it as well. Several of her finest poems originated or were completed in the nursing home, and she sent some of these to publishers. The same resilience of spirit also appears, after deep depression or silence, in her rousing a keen attention, again and again, to the life around her—to the condition and mannerisms of a roommate, other patients and their visitors, the chaplains; to the kindness of a nurse; or to music, a book review, certain phenomena of nature (the flowers, birds, trees, and good weather in which she finds increasing pleasure).

Some of these prevailing resurgences are apparently unwilled, as can be sampled in a few selections from the chronicle:

> September 8, 1975: (Having consigned myself to the grave, and not frivolously, I find myself quite interested in an illustrated article in color on Limoges enamels.)

> October 16, 1975: This time I wanted a kind of babes-in-the-wood death, with the leaves drifting down. I never saw them fall more gently.... I thought of "Call for the robin redbreast and the wren," which I took to be a sign I didn't want to die that minute.

> April 29, 1976: I do not know why the decomposition of speech and reason interests me, when it should appall me. I suppose because even now I am interested in putting things together....

We may suppose that her liberally trained sensitivity to the details and varieties of human life and art, together with her determination to be accurate and honest, makes Joyce Horner's pains and disappointments, as well as her delights, deeper, more keenly felt. Her long devotion to literature and music has, by now, become integral to her personality; thus we find everywhere in the chronicle quite natural allusions to the tradition, as to Webster's Jacobean play, quoted just above. Or take the occasion when, feeling very depressed and seeing two crows or blackbirds outside, she comments simply, "Twa corbies"—alluding to the old Scots ballad in which two such predatory birds consider the solitary corpse of a nameless knight far beyond human attention or even neglect. Now, there is considerable wit involved, of course, in making apt allusions when expressing feelings; such feats of association, simply as accomplishments of mind, can take away some of the sting in experience; they have the value, moreover, of generalizing one's private sensibility, evoking (paradoxically, in this case) the conviction of being not completely alone with such feelings in this life and in human history. So her beloved Shakespeare, Donne, and Keats among writers, as well as Bach, Mozart, and Beethoven among composers seem to be with her, sharing their experience and wisdom, through all her confinement.

We may also suppose that beyond the personal therapy which her chronicle afforded Joyce Horner during this period of serious confrontation with mortality is her desire to share the encounter with others for whatever values and wisdom might emerge in her presentation of the experience. "How, indeed," most of us must begin to ask in late middle age (if not earlier), "may I face the certain end of my earthly human awareness?" In reading Joyce Horner's chronicle, we may be heartened by her thoroughgoing gallantry as well as by her resilience of spirit, and I think we can trust that, though modest and tactful, she also rejoiced in her rich inner resources. She rates self-pity "low in the scale of emotions," and, as one who herself carries some light, she quotes with favor from John Donne, "I thank him who brings me a candle . . . when my sight grows old."

I have asked myself, as one also interested in composition, how Joyce Horner manages so effectively to sustain a public interest (a stranger's—my own, for example, as reader—for I never met her) in these originally private jottings. As suggested above, there is, no doubt, for anyone in late middle age a natural curiosity about her situation, but she can depend also on most adults' interest in the texture of another's expression of experience, the particular movements of someone else's mind: what will flow next, unexpectedly or otherwise, from any present thought and feeling? In this chronicle the unique, often allusive, movement of Joyce Horner's mind is unfailingly presented in a use of language that enables the unexpected with its initial surprise to seem natural and frequently delightful, so that we are spared too private or obscure a texture or style; as players of the role given by the script, we wouldn't feel at all awkward, uneasy, or self-conscious when performing it aloud in company or on a public stage. Often enough we may feel great satisfaction and, finally, even privilege.

Beyond the immediate textures sustaining our interest in the chronicle, there are various characterizations of patients and others which we follow as they develop, often over several months. There are themes, too, which recur: concern with the management of the nursing home, assessments of political figures and events, a continuing interest in the values of literature, music, art, and a consideration of philosophic and religious approaches to the great mysteries. There is even a delightfully sustained detestation and loathing of various commercial advertisements and the outrageous "Me-*Me*-ME!-ism" promoted by the popular-song industry for a susceptible market. As in a novel, all these developments as facets of the main one—how Joyce Horner, a fellow human being, confronts dissolution in old age—capture our interest and keep us reading.

Joyce Horner came to believe that she could never produce one particular poem she would have liked to compose—on the Body and the Soul—because she felt too close to it, was *living* it, and its ongoing, complex dailyness would not stop to be adequately grasped. The whole chronicle could be regarded as notes for that poem, I suppose. On October 5, 1976, while she was still thinking of writing the poem in a lyrical form, she anticipated its conclusion: "I'd like to end with waking to the pagan sun all over the window and the thrust of a young tree in spring." Even so, amen. That is also as good a wish as this reader can find for the final effect of Joyce Horner's chronicle and its best poems upon her readers.

Robert Tucker
Amherst, Massachusetts
September 1981

1975

March 11

Everyone wants to go home. Perhaps that says too much. Everyone "wants out." Or there may be some who are beyond wanting as much as that. But the woman who calls "Martha" over and over, the woman who calls "Eileen," want what they used to have and sometimes think they can get it if they call loud enough. (The woman who calls "Eileen" or "Irene" sometimes wants less than that. She wants someone to untie her and asks anyone who passes. Sometimes she'll say "Man, bring a hammer," but it's still to be untied. I wonder if she ever contemplates the next step after being untied; if she can.) As I write I hear a man across the hall say, "I couldn't go anywhere. I don't know where my folks are. I know where they were." That is the situation of many. One of the men in the room opposite owns a house quite near and it is empty, except for a cat whom his sister feeds. His roommate, who is 92 and very ready to be "going on 93," is as nearly reconciled as anyone I have met, the last of his family and with a certain pride in survival, in his able-bodiedness (he can take quite long walks in the right weather) in his appetite. He is deaf and cannot see to read, facts probably overlooked by people like me who think "if I could walk like that, I'd go home."

March 12

If I get outside, no one will ask me to lecture—from my Narrow Adult wheelchair—on Age or on non-scandalous nursing homes. I read in the *Times* that Susan Ford is keeping a diary as a good discipline and as the substance of a column for *Seventeen*. (She *is* 17.) I do not think *Modern Maturity* will offer me a contract. Like the *Reader's Digest* they prefer success and achievement, septuagenarian tennis, octogenarian dancing, and so on. Retired people standing on their heads—do you think at your age it is right? Heaven knows I am deeply indebted to the AARP, which keeps me going here, and I consider their factual newsletter useful; but *Modern Maturity* is not a publication one can read. I do not think this is envy of the nonagenarians who take headers into swimming pools in California. I do not *think* so.

In any case I am not keeping a journal as a discipline like Susan Ford, and, as I remember, Edward VI.

March 13

My next door neighbor appeared suddenly and asked me to turn down my radio—*Morning Pro Musica*, which is one of my principal consolations here, from the moment they take away my breakfast tray to the time I get up. I said yes, of course I'd turn it down but hadn't thought it was loud enough to penetrate to the next room. (I may have thought also that no one could object to Mozart coming softly through the walls.) She said, "Oh, yes. Don't you notice the noise the toilet makes when it flushes?"

Today when I was walking with my walker in the corridor, I observed a man on the arm of a nurse suddenly push her away, quite violently. Others have told me of having their hair pulled or faces slapped. Perhaps the staff has to be young. I am continually astonished at their willingness and patience, sometimes goodness. They do what I would have run away from at their ages, and long after. (The last time I went to see my mother, I began to run as soon as I got out of the house.) Perhaps they run when they come to the end of their eight-hour shift. Perhaps I exaggerate their heroism and idealism in easing the lot of the ill, disabled, lost, and incontinent, and perhaps they did not choose it but took it because it was a job.

Even so I praise them in the morning and in the afternoon and in the night watches.

March 16

A voice somewhere near cries out "Charlie, Charlie, Charlie," and "I can't get out" (Sterne—Marie Bertram in the "wilderness"). Then, "Charlie—if you'll get me out, I'll never bother you again." Then she runs through a list, Martha, Joanna, Mr. Moore, etc., etc., relatives, friends, neighbors. None of them come.

March 17

St. Patrick's. People wear shamrocks cut out of felt. There is a pie made of lime-green gelatine with whipped pseudo-cream. Even *Morning Pro Musica* failed me after nine o'clock and devoted the rest of the morning to Irish music of which there is very little so far as I can see. What we got were folk songs, not identified because Mr. Lurtsema could not read the labels which were in Irish. What I missed, when I had to get washed, was perhaps "Oft in the stilly night" or "I dreamt that I dwelt." I wonder why the Irish have created so little music. Because there was only one center and no patrons? (I am reading a life of Mozart.)

Thinking of Dick and Jimmy, who are critical of their jobs for different reasons, partly because they are different ages and different people. (Dick is not so critical as J. is at all—feels inadequate, rather.) Jimmy, who looks back to the old days in the old building, feels he has too many hard cases to get his work done. He was a navy nurse and detests sloppiness. ("What do you do with your clothes?" I heard him say to one patient, "You look like an unmade bed.") This morning I heard him say, "Where do you think you're going, Mr. A.? You haven't any pants on."

March 18

Avoided a St. Patrick's Day party yesterday. To come back to Jimmy. He is in his forties, a little grizzled, straight and foursquare. He treads the halls with the air of a man at home in the world. I am sure he is a pillar of the community and would be in the volunteer fire brigade, if he weren't in the ambulance corps. He whistles when he comes on in a morning and this is one of the sounds I am glad to hear. He delights in puns, which are often the same ones but that hardly matters. He defends himself from his job by language. One morning after an old Polish woman next door to us had been crying out all night, sometimes in Polish, sometimes in meaningless syllables (not that I understand any Polish at all, but I mean meaningless to Poles) and was still keeping it up with surprising energy when Jimmy brought in our breakfast trays, he said, "Pay no attention to the yelling, it's a recording." (We all defend ourselves.) I would be glad to see Jimmy coming in any emergency, smiling or even not smiling.

March 19

"And all the wheels of being slow." One of the bad days that may not recover, though the sun is coming out. It began with a bath for Mrs. R. and that upsets not only her. She has the never-smile-again look, so I say little. Then something happened to *Morning Pro Musica*—the station was dead—and I felt deserted, stranded under my blanket. I couldn't rise to the charity of thinking of all the people in pain and in the wilderness. The woman two doors up was calling for Gertrude and Mrs. Ryan, among others, to take the baby. I heard a nurse say, "Sweetheart, you haven't got a baby." But I didn't care, only felt I ought to. This was different when I first came from the hospital.

March 20

Wheels of being a bit faster today, after a bath, in which I luxuriate—would love to stay and luxuriate longer. Dreamed of Evelyn—she was bringing a whole crowd of Smith people to meet me, including Miss Hanscom (dead how many years?). There was something wrong, in that I was in a position I couldn't get down from, but it was better than the wandering-about-cities dream, which ends always with the realization, "But I can't walk."

To return to yesterday. It was different when I first came here, partly because I was in more physical discomfort, but partly too that I had never encountered, except by one and one, the pains of aging. In the hospital I had heard people cry out, but rarely. It was quiet at night. The halls were dark. The nurses came silently with flashlights. I did once see an old woman weeping uncontrollably and someone wheeled her away. But I was never anywhere before where so many cried out (it is not Bedlam and there is no one in the rooms near me who does) and at times I have felt almost annihilated by it—world sorrow, but in a small square of Massachusetts, hardly on the map except the geodetic survey maps we brought here when I began going out in a car. I know things I hadn't known before. (The woman who goes through all the people she has known, "Grandpa," "Mr. Martin," "Susie," is now saying, "I'll pay you. I'll be nice to you. I'll buy you a shirt." If they let her out. Her chronology is like dream-time.) I feel them in my bones and in my viscera.

March 23

Palm Sunday. The St. Luke's Passion which I never heard before and which I understand may not be by Bach, though it has some of the chorales in it—also *Nun Danket* which I love. It was my favorite hymn in the Guiseley School hymn book. I did exercises to it, thinking of the battle between body and soul that is always going on here and in which exercises to Bach seem to me one of the more benign phases—hardly a battle at all. In fact I am not sure it's the soul, but it *is* the moment and eternity. That is, eternity, in so far as I can conceive of it. If I say "so far as I can conceive it," I suppose I ruin the idea of eternity.

We have no palms for Palm Sunday, nor olive leaves as in Rome. (When I was a child I thought the palm willow, which we did not call pussy willow in Yorkshire, *was* palm and that it had been strewn on the way to Jerusalem.) But we have begun decorating for Easter, in the usual cute, but I dare say cheerful fashion—little figures coming out of church, just as we had figures round a table for Thanksgiving. There are Easter bunnies pasted here and there and I have always rejected the Easter bunny as a low, commercial form of the supernatural. There were no Easter bunnies in England when I was young but now even Fortnum & Mason catalogues have them. Mrs. R. has remarked that she'd rather see the money spent on decoration spent on food and I agree—except that if I knew all, I possibly would want it spent on the nurses' salaries or the cleaners' or the kind kitchen women who bring us trays.

Yesterday I was home.

(A long interruption for walk, rest—to the distant strains of the Holyoke parade on TV. St. Patrick, the South Hadley High School band—and then a curious apparition at the door, a short squat woman with grey hair sticking out round her head. She said, "Do you know who I am?" She looked like a witch. Then she went on and a moment later there was a scuffle in the corridor as one of the nurses tried to take her back to her room. It's curious, when I woke this morning I heard a high strange voice in the next room, a new voice, and thought "like a witch." Later I decided it was the witch in *Hansel and Gretel*, not *Macbeth*. And then there she was.

I was home and felt I was a lot of trouble and perhaps not worth it. That it was lovely to be at home, with crocuses coming up and purple finches and a fire and *The Marriage of Figaro* and, most, being with friends. But I am a liability and a millstone and I feel I'll get to be more of one, always taking and always asking for things. I laugh more when I'm at home than I get any occasion for here, and cry more here—though I don't think anyone knows—than anywhere I've ever been in my life. One nurse said, "Joyce is always cheerful."

March 24

Visit from Dr. Brewster, which has roused me—not for anything he said or did—to a kind of desperate energy. I feel I *will* get out, yet can't put on my own shoes. To be held because one can't put on one's own shoes and can't stand without them. At the moment, where is my lauded patience? I am miles from inheriting the kingdom of heaven and don't even want to. I want to go home, and I still know vividly what I mean by home, not what it was but what it is—a place of good lines, cheap furniture, old-shoe comfort, familiarity, love. (The woman up the corridor still crying "let me out" as monotonously as the starling, but varying only the names, must have only a dim image of home by this time. Perhaps some have none.)

The witch broke in on us last night through the bathroom door—the bathroom being between our room and hers. We locked the door on this side and she managed to unlock it and stuck her head in again. I found it unnerving but also funny. The young man who finally got her in bed had to defend himself. I believe she would scratch and bite. She has a peculiarly high-pitched scream. There is something formidable about her. Charles Addams—it has suddenly come to me that she reminds me of the Charles Addams's man, not the woman. I should feel pity, but I can't. But she wants to get out too and even tried to last night through the door at the end of the corridor. The man in the corner room said he wished she'd got away.

I said I cried more here and it is true but half my tears are literary. I find myself thinking, "If ever thou gavest hosen, and shoon. . . . / Sit thee down and put them on" (this partly, I am sure because of my preoccupation with the shoes I can't put on) and weeping because I thought I wouldn't qualify and because I love the poem.

March 25

Ave verum corpus on the radio, played three times over in different versions, almost overwhelming. R. Lurtsema said if they'd had twenty versions he would have played them and I felt I could have listened to twenty. (The death in the world today is King Feisal's and in this hospital, Mrs. C's.) I did not know, because I haven't got there yet in the biography, that it was written near the end of Mozart's life. Thinking of stone walls, etc., and fishes that tipple in the deep, as I often have here because of the universal desire to be out, I believe my *freest* moments have been spent listening to the *Morning Pro Musica*. They are not happier than the visits of friends but freer, uncluttered (unless they come and try to wash me) by practical necessities and plans and moving objects from one place to another. It is the time that it is easiest to forget the body, and the clamorous ego that will get into poetry. I expect if you're tethered to a chair or nailed down by pain in bed, these badly insulated cement walls *do* a prison make.

On the matter of getting washed versus *Morning Pro Musica*, I felt the race most in the St. John Passion when I found myself thinking as time went on, "Please (God!) don't let them come before 'Es ist vollbracht' and not before 'Ruhe Wohl.' " I got my wish. (I remember the wholly satisfying performance at St. Bartholomew's the Great, with Peter Pears as the Evangelist, Janet Baker, and Benjamin Britten in the audience, and the woman next to me following the score with tears running down her cheeks.) I am ashamed that thinking of "stone walls," etc., it was at least three minutes before I could think of either Lovelace's name or the first line. There, day by day, flake by flake, goes my own education and my education of others.

March 26

They moved the witch yesterday and I am hard-hearted enough not to care where they moved her to. I am thankful for the roommate who had to endure her, though briefly, after a long dose of Mrs. McD.'s cheerful, garrulous nuttiness. She said today, "I'm so glad to have someone rational." So now this corner should be quiet, even though *rational* may overstate the collective mental state of these six rooms. (I can hear the nurse who is feeding the woman up the hall who calls out to all the people she has ever known, "The babies are all grown up, Mary.")

I think of the people who have written books in prison—Boethius, Raleigh, Bunyan, and lately, I shouldn't be surprised, Jeb Stuart Magruder or John Dean. The two last and their like may cash in on them, but I don't suppose they'll be about prison any more than *Pilgrim's Progress* or *The History of the World* is. And this isn't prison, except for the drab rooms, with nothing but grey, white, and tan and their narrow space suggesting cells to one who has never been in a cell. (And we can't get out.) It makes me wish I could write a book, or what I'd really like here of all things—poems—even one poem ("committed linnets"). But I haven't a hope. My range of words diminishes—it's hardly up to crossword strength—and I no longer think in images. I am puzzled why the power of image-making should leave one, but it left me long before I got in here. I haven't even the desire to write a novel. (There is a story in this week's *New Yorker* about a daughter helping her mother with a crossword puzzle and I thought of how I helped mine—except that she was just as good as I was—and that it was

one of the things that brought us together in her old age, that
and sitting on a seat on the seafront and watching the people
passing or sitting over a cup of tea, anywhere. But I failed as a
daughter.)

> Teach us to care and not to care
> Teach us to sit still.

In spite of everything, a very good day.

March 27

Too extroverted. Too long at the hairdresser's. Too little exercise. The hairdresser is silver-blonde, by whatever means; capable of great speed, highly competent in moving us crocks from
chair to chair. Critical of the permanent wave Millie came all this
way to give me. Exercises professional charm. Greek Orthodox?

The woman up the hall, going through her litany of names,
called "Joyce" and I felt summoned. They say she has a very sweet
smile. One nurse told me, "She is the sort of person who ought
to be surrounded with babies." When I see her, she is always in
distress, tied, in the doorway. Not looking at all like Spenser's
charity.

March 28

Good Friday. There was no mass, as I'd been told there was
going to be, and as an onlooker I felt disappointed in not seeing
the priest sweep down the corridor with his acolytes and candles,
ringing his bell. (The same handbell was used by Santa Claus, and
my roommate, who receives mass, said: "Good God, is it the
priest?") He brings a bit of ceremony into these unceremonial
halls. For some, I am sure, he brings comfort, though he is not to
me a sympathetic person. One day when he brought the mass to
Mrs. R. and to whatever he said she responded, "Oh, Lamb of
God that ———." The priest said, "Stop talking and open your
mouth." Without belief, I find the "Lamb of God"—what is it,
petition, ejaculation, cry?—terribly moving at all times, in English
or Latin. I don't think it is just literariness. It is at least half "if it

were possible." Meanwhile the sins of the world accumulate in frightening fashion.

Today there was fish to fast on and apple pie to cancel the effect.

Reading *Country Life*, the Christmas number—which is where I am, between the slowness of sea mail and my late start on anything of that size and weight—I find myself delighting in its bits of miscellaneous information (e.g., that the *cosset* lamb, because it grew up following the shepherd, often became the bellwether) along with its visual appeal (in that particular article magnificent reproductions of shepherds at Bethlehem. . . .) and its invitations to nostalgia for the past. When I was a child I looked at auctioneers' catalogues and thought of the houses I'd like to live in. Now I go lightly over the advertisements of houses to be sold at auction or by private treaty, stopping mainly over the rivers I'd never heard of. There is only one house I want to live in. As for the beautiful objects, China jars, etc., tankards, even Sheraton chests of drawers, I like to see them and to think I never had and never will have them, am glad they exist and have long stopped wanting them, except of course that I could sell them and pay a nurse at night and go home.

Nice fable written by Mozart to his cousin about the shepherd who had to get eleven thousand sheep across a narrow bridge —this seems my day for sheep. To think of his seeing himself in terms of eleven thousand. Quantity and genius. Another nice thing about the shepherd was that he had a stick with a fine red ribbon in his hand. Mozart.

I heard the witch say—when a nurse was wheeling her in a wheelchair past our door and had said, "Let's go and see your friends down here"—"I haven't any friends." The nurse said, "You'd have more friends if you didn't hit so many people." Then somehow the nurse must have effected a change, at least for the moment. From the end of the corridor I heard the witch singing.

March 29

Grey, sleepy. Few visitors because they will, many of them, come tomorrow, often to pick up their relatives and take them home to dinner. Most of the people here are much visited. They are not the deserted, forgotten people of the scandalous nursing homes in the Nader reports or the *New York Times*. There was one man who came every day to see his sister and took home her nightgown to wash. He used to call on several people, including us, and I imagined the place made a center of social life for him. He was a retired nurse, but he has not been back since her death last week. I noted in the paper that his father had one of the typical French Canadian names—Midard—that are dying out every day. The *Holyoke Transcript* will soon have no more Adelards, Trofimes, Severes, even Napoleons.

April 1

Although there are robins, I come back from Easter at home in a state of deep depression. Usually I have felt safe coming back, and perhaps welcome.

April 2

At this point I was put to bed, where writing ends. But the depression was there again when I woke this morning, as after my three-day visit, I feel I have lost hope of going home. The obstacles remain so great, and there's not even the possibility of staying here if I become "custodial care"—the insurance company is sniffing around already. But I will not write out of self-pity, which I place very low in the scale of emotions—even nostalgia ranks higher, its imagery is more varied.

Mrs. McD. has gone, they say to a place where she can have a room to herself, though rumors differ as to the place. She should have a room of her own. We got her only in passing, when she'd pause at the door to tell us what all the people eating in the solarium had on their trays and, once, how she helped the kitchen people by gathering all the paper cups together after the meal and putting them one inside another. But her roommate got an interminable flow and, she tells me, was once wakened at 3 A.M. to have Browning read to her. And after that, the witch, though for only two nights.

Finished W. J. Turner on Mozart yesterday, with the pangs I've had many times for his end. But I do not agree with W.J.T.

11

that the kind of genius Mozart had and Shakespeare had is the love of God. A godlike love of man, perhaps. W.J.T. makes a great point of its including tragedy and comedy. But the love of God must transcend tragedy and comedy. (Are the terrible sonnets tragic? I'd say not or rather it isn't the love of God that makes them tragic—"my cries heave, herds-long," etc. It's the loss of God. I suppose it might be argued that the loss depends on the love —"But worse" because the lost don't care. But the "come under my cloak" seems to me like human tragedy. That is why I do not see how there can be an omniscient and caring God who nevertheless lives in bliss. Milton gets himself into this dilemma when the angels after the fall have only as much pity as is compatible with bliss. And if there is a God, he must be omniscient or there is no point in him. End parenthesis.)

Except that it has just struck me, since supper, that Milton's omniscient God talking about his omniscience is so much less sympathetic than the power that made the world in Book VII. Or is it the world he made that is sympathetic?

Completely unrelated note on Gerald Ford—bells don't *toll* for freedom. Like Richard Glenn Gettell, he'd better keep off literary allusions—as R.G.G. wisely did.

April 3

Now the witch is crying, "Help me out" in her characteristic high, piercing tones but when I passed the door on my walker ten minutes ago she was quiet, crooning a reminiscent spell. I hear she is leaving us for which we all feel relief, without allowing ourselves to think of the people where she is going. Or of her. . . . I think of saints and priests I've read of, and the one Bertile knows in Baltimore, who do not discriminate in their love. She'd hit them too and it would not change them.

Listening to conversations between patients, one is struck by the smallness of the circle. Northampton, Southampton, Easthampton, Westhampton, Williamsburg, Goshen. "My brother lived on State Street, next door to ———." This is the most provincial society I've lived in since I was a child, when everybody knew everybody in Lofthouse and Robin Hood. Not that this is exactly a society, perhaps not even a community, as Mount Holyoke College is, but it is local and fairly homogeneous—not a black face to be seen, some Canadian French and some Polish spoken as in all this region, especially among the old, and not much evidence, except among the nurses, of interests beyond the personal. It is, as far as I can see, classless, and looking back on my first ten years in Lofthouse I feel there was little class distinction there that was obvious to a child. (I did hear the words "no class" spoken of such a one, from time to time. Also "gentry," etc.) One of the "great" houses stood unoccupied, then was used by the manager (from London, and so suspect) of the ill-fated Lofthouse Park about which I once wanted to write a children's book. The Andrews family from London was one of my first glimpses of a world beyond. They kept a boy in buttons, but did not, I believe, pay their debts. They did not last long. The other house, Lofthouse Hall, belonged to an explorer who was hardly ever there. No one in the village went away to boarding school. But then everywhere was more provincial, especially perhaps in the north. This is almost opposite from the academic world and the Idea of a University.

Notice—that the price of a room has been put up $2.00 a day.

Curtains, the kind drawn for decency and privacy, taken down, washed, and returned within a few hours. Everything is washed, mopped, polished as on the Cunard ships I used to cross in. Whatever one can say about the place, it is what my grandmother used to call "bottom clean."

Something I liked in the *National Trust* report, said of Sir Robert Shirley (when?) who built the church of Staunton Harold (where?): "whose singular praise it is to have done the best things in ye worst times and hoped them in the most callamitous." Seventeenth century? Sixteenth?

April 4

Cold, bursts of sun, snow flurries, a wind, but better than the flooding rain of yesterday. They say the little Mill River we saw in our fall excursions moving gently over stones is now high, brown, and angry.

Mr. Drake came in this morning to talk to Mrs. R. I have

thought of him before as without any human feelings—I have hardly spoken to him, only seen him stalking the corridors without a smile or the possibility of a smile. But he was gentle with her and humored her when she said she hoped the new building that was going on (here) was not encroaching on anyone else's land as she had only thirty-five feet (five miles away) and her driveway was only so wide.

She has spent the afternoon, since the visit of her son, in anger at the thought of the loss of her things, household goods. Her children have divided and taken the spoil. (A situation which has recurred in my life so often, but never quite in these circumstances. Not that I know the circumstances exactly as they appear to her.) She grew angrier as she thought of more things—"my silver dish, my stainless steel knives—who got this?" she asked her son over and over. He had some, but not the best. Perhaps anger keeps one from self-pity. In any case I am not going to feel superior to her because even if I don't worry about *things,* I do about money and do paltry sums in my head, always ending in the impasse that I can neither go home nor stay here long. Living with a blind person in itself might be enough to stop one's pluming oneself on anything. It ought to be.

April 5

Mrs. R. still murmuring about silver and steak knives, but more plaintively than anything. A cold, grey day, but still. We had a tough nurse this morning from another wing, the only one of her kind I've encountered here. When she'd wrenched my knees enough, trying to put my shoes on, she called Jimmy, who put them on as if he'd been in a shoe shop all his life, painlessly and without a shoe horn. (Just a little while ago, when we were eating our nasty lunch, I heard someone yelling, "Jimmy, come quick, the new man's choking.")

Speaking of toughness in nurses, I thought they were all so when I first came from the hospital. That was partly a general feeling of disorientation after having been thrown out so quickly, partly that they said, "What's the matter?" when you rang the bell —and my terrible difficulties with ringing these bells—instead of, "Can I help you?" as in the Cooley-Dickinson, partly that they shouted to each other more in the corridors, often about bedpans and commodes (the old). And there was one I am now very fond of who came in the first day and said, "Come on. Get up for supper. We don't have people laying around in bed, here." But now there is almost no one I don't welcome and some I feel warmly attached to. Some I have regretted deeply when they left. I can see, too, that they have to develop a different manner with the old, many of them deaf, many far advanced into senility. "While we are *still decaying*—." I used to think that a poor thing to say to Corinna and even that he'd used up all his other rhymes for *maying,* though the stanza is magnificent. But now I feel let us go, not a-maying—but go where we can in November, maybe December, while we are still decaying. For instance, if I'm asked, I'll go home tomorrow.

Mrs. R. says, "I had a quadruple-plated pitcher. . . ."

My roughneck nurse this morning remarked of the radio music (Posthorn Serenade), "That's nice music. Kind of soothing. It isn't trying to tell you something, like most music." By that I suppose she means it isn't saying, "Tie a yellow ribbon round the great oak tree," or "I won't last a day without you," or "I'm a hell of a woman and I'll make you a hell of a man." I've had an unprecedented opportunity to hear the words of popular songs here—not since my dancing days have I paid any attention to them. Some themes remain the same—"I'm blue without you." But there are far more songs of separation (real separation, not just "all alone feeling blue")—"it's all over," "I'm going crazy," "it couldn't last." And the man in "Tie a yellow ribbon" had been in prison and one I heard the other night began "I'm drinking again." But I liked the idea that Mozart was nice and soothing because he wasn't trying to tell you anything. Maybe I'll end up liking her too.

April 9

After three days at home and more mixed feelings than I can chronicle. April still cold, but today there is no snow. At home read (because that's where the reading group had arrived) the Struldbrugs chapter without feeling I was living among them. They aren't Struldbrugs and I am not. Even Mrs. B. aged 107 had the energy to kick me when I was waiting in line (wheelchair line) in front of her to see the foot doctor. On the other hand I read "Stay with me Ariel while I pack" with strong, partly self-pitying emotion but I insist partly not. We must read some of Auden aloud next time I go home, for go home I will even though I come back lame as a tree, as my mother used to say. I understand it now, your legs can feel like trees, young birches, I think. Like some of these out here. I wonder about the end of the song to Ariel "as . . . we take the silent passage into discomfort." It seems rather the discomfortable passage into silence. But Auden didn't believe that, so the silence must be the no-longer-singing passage into the uncomfortable, uncomforted, beyond-comfort preliminaries of death. There may be an element of the Stoic's silence too. Lord, I sound as if I were teaching a class.

April 10

The witch is gone and Mrs. Martha Danielson who runs through her string of names is muted today. I was aware of her only when I was passing the door. I am told she has a daughter who comes to see her every day.

Yesterday bell ringers to entertain us in the Happy Room. (I am told it was a patient who suggested the name, so one can't blame the Activities woman who runs the festival dinners and the so-called concerts.) I did not go and by now they have stopped putting pressure on me and on Mrs. R. I may miss good things but I didn't want to hear tunes played on handbells, even if they'd been by superstars. (The one time I liked handbells was up in the tower of Winchester Cathedral hundreds of years ago it seems, when we went up with a remarkably knowledgeable verger [Adams?] who gave us each a handbell—we were in the room right under the bells—and pointed to us in turn to make us play a peal.) I have questioned the wisdom of these Happy Room functions because they surround one with the threats of age and decay one wishes to forget, or at least not intensify—a circle of mirrors, glances into possibility. Death sitting at the table in all his bones would not appall me in the same way. I don't think anyone old is *afraid* of death, though many, including Mrs. B., who will be 108 on Monday, may want life to go on. But I am told that a good many people like these things in the Happy Room—our late Mrs. McD. was one of them—and therefore Activities are a good thing. If I say "for some people," I sound condescending, and when I go to the things I note an element of condescension in my putting in an appearance which I dislike and struggle against, as against so many things. I still feel, however, that a number of people are there just because they're put in chairs and taken—those who go to sleep, those who have to be fed, those who don't even know they are there.

Today I feel I can hardly bear it to be so far into April and no nearer home.

I did not listen to the President last night. I watch the political programs less, though I still watch the news and *Washington Week*. This is partly because I know Mrs. R. does not care for the TV, unless it is a musical program, but partly too that I've no one to comment to as it's going on. It is the same with the *Times*—I don't enjoy it so much when we can't read the editorials aloud, though Elizabeth keeps all the good ones for me.

(The voice of Mrs. Sullivan at the other end of the corridor is audibly calling, "Martha, Martha" as ever; she never changes her note. Once she was next door and it was very loud. *Martha* happens to be the name of Mrs. Danielson, who also calls such a variety of names of both sexes and who just now is calling "Kathleen," which is Mrs. Sullivan's name. But they don't want one another.)

To return to TV, I enjoyed so much at home being able to see "Behind the Lines," for instance, and tolerated an interview with Clarence Kelley of the FBI, who has no jargon if very few words, because we could laugh. When I am with Elizabeth, I feel more world indignation too. Though even here alone, I have risen to the act of writing to my congressman. And I feel useless pangs over the Vietnamese and Cambodians, so many streaming along the roads, and wonder if I can send a little more to this or that relief society, and then wonder what I have and how my insurance will hold up and what happens next.

But as I have just been presented by a kind lady with the *New Republic*, so back into the fray. (And I see that T.R.B. begins his lead editorial with "Hey nonny nonny" which cheers me.)

T.R.B.: ". . . the moral dilemma between compassion and arithmetic." The nation's, the Congress's, millions of people's, mine. Only the saints are exempt from it.

Have just discovered that officially they call the nurses' station "the Care Area"—the nurse who told me said she asked, "Where's that?" Even here, where spades are on the whole called spades, that sort of language intrudes itself.

April 11

Reread Elsie's letter and was pleased by the fact that at the very lowest tides—and these were the lowest of the century—the Jerseyites (or do they call themselves Jerseyaises—I think perhaps Jerseyais is just the language) go out to look for the lost manor of St. Ouen, called La Brequette. It's like the beginning of a story, but probably a children's story. The facts end there, as they found nothing, except hundreds of ormers which Elsie describes as a rather dull shellfish, not worth the trouble, but much loved by the natives.

Our Protestant chaplain came in to say goodbye yesterday before he sets off to England to visit places connected with John Wesley, also to buy himself a waistcoat. It is good of him to spend so much time calling on a lost soul and an R.C., but he prays for us, with immense adaptability to circumstance (I suppose that's the point of extempore prayers, though I prefer "Lighten our darkness," etc.). Actually I am moved that the Rev. Mr. Montgomery should bother to pray for me and sometimes I admire his readiness, as at the time when we'd been complaining about the food and he said, "Remember the words of St. Paul: 'Teach us when to abound and when to be abased.' " He never preaches to us, like my first hospital religious visitor, the lady of the tracts who came and sat beside me in Leeds Infirmary in England, after I'd had my appendix out—in the long ward with the red blankets and the big fireplace at each end. She read to me the chapter about Nicodemus and went on to say, "Now you're like Nicodemus," and much more. That was when I was twenty.

Michael Arlen (Jr.) good on the way the TV shots of Vietnamese refugees fit too easily into our lives. Speaking of a *Times* headline "Indochina déjà vu," he says, "Ironies . . . provide a certain distance, or the semblance of perspective to someone trying to confront a wretched situation. But I doubt whether irony will be of much help to anyone now." That's where Auden was right in Prospero's—I can't quote it right: "Shall I be able to suffer without saying something ironical or funny about suffering?" There are depths and straits where irony is no defense. It returns with recovery.

Mrs. Danielson is now calling "Kathleen" at the top of her lungs, loud enough to reach the Kathleen who is calling "Martha." The wrong Kathleen and the wrong Martha. What kind of irony is that?

Walked on a small square of cement outside. Spring.

Evening, and a great fight is going on, two female voices and one male in the region of the Care Area. Voices raised in what sounds to be a mixture of English and Polish. Our next door neighbor says it is two daughters, visiting a father. Once one daughter said, "If you think we're coming every night when you. . . ."

April 12

Connie brought me *The Wide Wide World* which she picked up at a library sale and I spent a nostalgic hour over Ellen's buying the writing desk, etc. Now the facts in it interest me more, e.g., that one had, by that time, a choice between envelopes and having a blank page for the address. I was never moved by Ellen's tears even as a child, but I'd forgotten she let them drip into the basin as she was getting washed. Her chief rival for tears (I leave out Niobe) is, I think, Emily in *The Mysteries of Udolpho*.

Jo mentioned the line in "The Lotus-Eaters" as coming into his mind when he saw the devastation of Vietnam: "Clanging fights, and flaming towns, and sinking ships, and praying hands." So I got out "The Lotus-Eaters" and read it again. There isn't anything else so good in Tennyson, is there? But I forget I am released from asking that part of the question.

When Mrs. R. is reminiscent I enjoy her. The game parties, or suppers, I think they called them, in a hunting shack belonging to some ancient Hadley character, where they all took something—a pheasant, a rabbit, quail and sat on the floor to eat and drink. I

19

gather she had a sudden and rather brutal initiation into being a farmer's wife and this she remembers straight. Like the detail about the farm in *The Wide Wide World* which is better than H. B. Stowe to my mind, though the pious parts are much worse, worse than I remembered.

April 14

Somehow, in a blissful half-asleep condition before breakfast, found myself thinking of laughter—the kind of helpless laughter one does not get in age, though I still laugh—here with the nurses out of a kind of good fellowship on the absurdities of the body, or at least—this to myself—the *New Yorker* or Peter Lisagor. But one never dissolves in laughter as, for instance, Susan and George and I used to on our Sunday walks, making up a Walter poem as we went along, each adding a line or a couplet— the traditional situation of an uncle asking young men their intentions, our Cousin Mildred with all her suitors and our vague, nutty Aunt Edith, who all with the process of time became half-fictionalized and the situation a series of comic conventions. I suppose then we laughed at the essential comedy, at our feeling of cleverness in inventing a new variation on it, even at our rhymes, but also we were in the open air—on Chippenfield Common, perhaps, sitting on thyme or heather, eating and drinking, with the sun at least going in and out. (I'm not sure we made up any poems on the wet Sundays when the only "bright intervals" came in the train.) And we were in our twenties and thirties. We could go into fits, e.g., when Susan rhymed *calico* with *De Bello Gallico*—that was a poem about all the materials in Walter's warehouse. I remember it began, "Walter came home with a yard of madapolam" which places it in time, though I can't be sure what time except time past. Who's even heard of madapolam? (Who was it told Mother and me once that she'd had people rolling off their chairs with laughing? We used to quote her afterwards.)

A visit from a patient whose daughter comes to see her every day and who complains bitterly all the time. Mrs. R. worked really hard to try to cheer her up and I admired her. The daughter who gives up her time to push her about in a wheelchair can't have enjoyed her mother's remark that her husband had told her, "When

I go, you'll be alone. None of your children will look after you."
But I suppose that too is the mind going; the trouble is one can't
foresee the forms it may take. The daughter said to me *sotto voce*,
"she was always like that."
Ate my first bagel, made by one of the young nurses. Food.
Went to the 108th birthday party of Mrs. B.

April 15

A low day after a high one, so I'll go back to the birthday party which was partly good, partly terrible. The heroine of it com-
ported herself with great dignity and looked as if she knew all this
was in honor of her and accepted it. She sat in her chair like a
queen—she is rather the shape of Queen Victoria, larger. She
looks well, is no wrinkled hag—I have more wrinkles and she was
born before my mother. Around her and beside her sat the family,
five generations. She said nothing and did not smile until they put
the youngest great-great-grandchild on her lap. (I regret to say
they did this for the camera, one a TV camera.) Then when the
child cried she dandled it and sang: "O Danny Boy" to it, as from
long practice. I felt this represented one kind of success in life,
though in a nursing home. The bad part was the entertainment,
though the Rev. Mr. Montgomery says we must think of such
things as people doing their best. I might have been able to think
the woman who sang was at least a gallant performer, if I hadn't
been so hot and everything—her voice, the dreadful piano, the
drums—too loud. I was very glad to be delivered by friends' arriving from any more music and even from the birthday cake. The
woman who sang was evidently an old trouper. She wore black
satin with spangles (only probably that is old-fashioned language
for what she wore). She also told anecdotes in the pauses between
songs. The songs included "Let Me Call You Sweetheart," "A Bi-
cycle built for Two" and, of course, "Danny Boy." (We used to
sing "Oh Strength and Stay" to the Londonderry Air—was it
Guiseley School or at L.G.H.S?)
Yesterday saw or heard two things I liked. One a nurse talking to Mrs. Danielson to take her mind off the people who don't
come. "What is your favorite bird? What is your favorite flower?"
The other: the difficult, combative Mr. A. was standing in his

doorway, looking glum, and a nurse went up to him and said something in Polish, then sang a little Polish song to him and his face relaxed and his feet began to move as if he were dancing.

Being with the young (really young often—20, 21, 22) I sometimes feel old pedagogic stirrings. On Ash Wednesday when I saw so many people, old and young, marked with ashes on the forehead, I had a terrible desire to read "Ash Wednesday" aloud to someone. (Not to meditate on Ash Wednesday.) I once got as far as asking the superintendent of nurses whether there wasn't a blind person here I could read poetry to. She said: "I don't know about *poetry*. I'll look into it though." I am sure she's right. Not poetry. What Mrs. R. liked having read to her best was the account of Christina Onassis' inheritance. She also liked the chapters on Northampton in a book on Jenny Lind that was lent to me.

Can one be honest about anything but facts? And of those, just what one hears and sees?

April 16

Thinking of Mrs. Danielson who can always pull another name out of the hat. (She is calling "Mr. Cross" which is one I never heard before.) I also think how impossible it would be for me to hang on to all my names—all the lists I had to learn every semester and how there was always a period in which it seemed impossible I should learn them, and then suddenly they were all individuals, with their names fixed for a while. While one goes through the process of losing more and more, one is still startled when a name from the remote past—Canada or Hood College— comes into one's mind, with the image attached, and sometimes a whole scene, with words. The name *Mary Lyons Agnew* arrives from nowhere and I think of taking her home from church over the snow, and she leaning all her weight—considerable—on my arm. She could have grandchildren now. Not worth mentioning if one did not see or hear so many people who have lost their boundaries in time, place.

This morning the nice woman in the next room had a heart attack when my nurse had got one shoe and stocking on me in preparation for taking me to the bath. While I can't say I like staying in that state, I was impressed at the way they got to her and stayed with her. An hour and a half later, when I was walking (the Director of Nursing put my other shoe and stocking on), I met the original nurse coming out of the patient's room for the first time since she left me. Yesterday, too, they rallied around Mrs. R. in an emergency and saw her through, but today when I told her of Becky's staying in the next room an hour and a half she said, "And leave the rest of us to die."

April 19

The bicentennial of Paul Revere's ride, which will be re-enacted in Boston and in many of the subsidiary towns in Mass., including South Hadley, where the riding master will ride a horse around the green, and Curtis Smith (Biology) will fire a cannon, and then a ball will be held—Mary Benson says that is unhistorical. Here I am sure Mr. Drake will not get on a horse and ride around the green square in front, though this terrain would lend itself to riding.

Indoors I awoke to the pleasure of daffodils on the table, though they're drooping a little. I won't say they are my favorite flower, as I like too many (not all, not gladioli or amaryllis or . . .) but they are spring in a way nothing else is, not even the forerunners. Farndale, the Lakes, to say nothing of all the poetry. I won't say I have a favorite passage of poetry   that is even more impossible than the flowers—but the "O Proserpina" passage could be, almost, if one could set a passage against a whole poem or scene or play. It is just that it comes first to mind, like the voice of God speaking to Job which I might call my favorite passage in the Bible —or perhaps might have called would be nearer the truth. Perhaps I'd still call it the most thrilling, but I ought to be beyond the need of thrills. Visceral ones.

Mrs. R., who feels ill, roused herself nevertheless to a scene about changing her nightgown—much Jesus, Mary, Joseph, and God damn it, but "they" changed it nonetheless.

Have got into a delightful correspondence with a former student's daughter, the first of its kind, who has just this year gone up to Cambridge and is bringing back my freshman feelings, gowns, bicycles (which I dared not ride in Oxford) and the towpath at "Toggers," evensong—for her it's at King's, for me, Magdalen.

She said among other things she'd climbed a *stickle* near Kendal—that must be a Cumberland word, I'd never heard it before. She says her grandfather lived there and I remember she had one grandparent called *Cawkrodger*—utterly north country like my *Clough*. One of my Clough ancestors rode with fleeces in his saddlebags to Ulverston market and I take pleasure in that brief glimpse of him—less than a glimpse—as I do in Mary Crosland eloping in her red cloak or Grace Joyce Lake riding to church on a white horse. I wish I'd wanted to ask more about these people when there were people there to answer. At the time I thought Grandma Horner an awful bore when she talked to me about Grace Joyce Lake and hardly listened.

April 22

Home again. Awaiting me here was a letter from Jersey, with the essay by Elizabeth Cragoe about her farm, and I was so pleased with what she and Desmond are doing. They have cows and chickens mainly, I think, but the delightful thing is that they are trying to have as many wild flowers as possible, and planting them where they've been lost. She said she wanted it "painted all with variable flowers" and naturally that pleased me, along with the quotations from Shakespeare and M. Arnold. I felt really warm toward her. I hope she does write a book on her farm, *en fleur*.

April 23

Shakespeare's birthday and R. J. Lurtsema disappointed me in devoting so brief a time to it when there is so much he could have done. It also happened to be Prokofiev's birthday and we got, in my opinion, too much of him.

Nothing new here, except the wonderfulness of being able to step across the threshold with one's walker and walk up and down three cement blocks in the sun, a titmouse singing. Perhaps I have exhausted the possibilities of these sanitized halls and the evidences of mortality within my range of seeing and hearing.

When they took our washbowls to sterilize, Mrs. R. protested, being convinced that they would come back full of the germs that are running rampant in this place. But last night she told me the story of her painful childhood and here I think there is no fantasy. Her father emerges as the sympathetic, touching figure who taught her things like "The Midnight Ride of Paul Revere," but couldn't look after his family when his wife died. She was sent to an aunt, with one dress and no coat to her name. Later she was called home again when her father remarried, but there the stepmother tied her to a bedpost and whipped her; he sent her away again to another aunt, with one quarter in her pocket. Years later, when she was happily married (the second marriage), he turned up once to see her and afterwards sent her a black plush coat lined with red satin. She never saw him again. I should never judge her. She made me feel my childhood was spent in clover, though we were nobody.

Reading in a review in the *New Republic* about Chinese hospitals (*A Death with Dignity* by Lois Snow) about the greater humanness and humanity of Chinese doctors and nurses. The thing they describe—their staying with the family and "mingling helpfully" with them *is* different from anything here. But I find most of the people here both human and humane, familiar with the patients in a way that is different from that in hospitals proper—I include the man who waxes the hall and the people who bring us food. (The doctors hardly come into this, appearing rarely.) I feel uninhibited and free among them. One or two seem like students I know well. But I'm sure the Chinese don't put pressure on their patients to go to entertainments. If one got so many marks for going, or had a cutting system. . . . I am at this moment avoiding some dancers.

April 24

Mrs. R. in a grim mood last night and today. When she is angry her face narrows, nose and chin come nearer together and her dark eyes blaze. Last night she almost threw off sparks in a fury against the nurse who was putting her to bed—I don't think I knew then why, except that the wrong thing seemed to be said and then the curses flew. However weak she is, she can throw tremendous energy into her anger—or does anger supply the energy? Afterwards she fell into a less intense intermittent complaint against her children and the loss of her things. (A son and his wife had been to see her earlier and all was amicable and smiling.) Today, over the lunch tray (and it was abominable) she said she hoped they'd have to go to a nursing home some day and find out. Does she really hope it? I'd say no. She believes St. Anne de Beaupré could restore her sight.

Reading what seemed to me a remarkable review of a new edition of Dante (the edition by Charles Singleton, the review by D. S. Carne-Ross). It jumps with my state of mind. Of course I'd always been struck by the fact that it was hell where the ghosts wanted to know what was going on in Florence—I once tried to write a poem about the ghosts in the S. Hadley graveyard wanting to know, in the fall, what was going on now, now, today, but I never finished it—and I'd find it hard to accept what St. Augustine says in the passage Carne-Ross quotes: "Suppose we were wanderers in a strange country and could not live happily away from our fatherland . . . and wishing to put an end to our misery, determined to return home. . . . But the beauty of the country through which we pass, and the very pleasure of the motion, charm our hearts, and turning these things which we ought to use into objects of enjoyment, we become unwilling to hasten the end of our journey. . . . Such is a picture of our condition in this life of mortality."

(Interruption for a terrible scene between Mrs. R. and her daughter, with a sad ending, "I'd better take myself off as I'm sure you'd rather see Willy than me." I had to go on copying with tears, I hope no one saw. It is a circle of hell to be imprisoned by things and also by the love of one child above the others. When one has lost too much of one's memory to be fair or to care about the amenities. I can't be certain, of course, that it's all loss of memory, or even the loss of sight which must deliver one over more to one's obsessions, I don't know.)

To return to Dante, most of us don't want a heavenly home. As C-R says throughout, we can't take over his terms, or even desire permanence. (As I write this I hear a man in the hall say, "I can't go home. They won't have me. They've put me here.") But I still feel it is the disappearance of God in the world at large that has piled up the mountain of crime—rape, murder, theft, arson every day. But Mrs. R. believes in God. . . . And of course he's

(C-R) right: poetry, most of it, celebrates transitory joy. And when we are young, "face downwards in the sun," we exult in transience itself. Though I still feel shaken, I ate the apple pie that Mrs. R.'s daughter brought me and noted—I'd wondered about it—that she ate hers too. It was good, however transitory. We spoke about it after a long silence. She even bragged of it to the tray-pickerup.

April 25

Sequel to the above scene last evening, when W. and his wife arrived and Mrs. R. gave her account of what had happened, "Irene got mad and went off in a huff." Much of what she remembered had enough truth in it to make one sure she wasn't being dishonest but only remembering bits out of context. All terribly unfair and perhaps unfairness rouses me more than some worse things. I can't be sure that all the unfairness is a result of loss of memory (among other things she said was, "My mind is as clear as a bell"). Willy was always the favorite son. I might have had favorites, if I'd had children, as of course I had favorite students but I hope I didn't show it. Loss of memory in Miss Snell, so long as she was conscious of it, made her anxious and worried but it didn't make her put all the blame on other people. When she reached the stage of having forgotten she'd lost it, she was amiable and kept something of her old response to people without knowing quite who they were. She had very few images left—an incident in childhood, the opening of college and her new freshman class. I think Mrs. R. is at the stage in which she is anxious to insist that her mind is clear, and that *she* remembers what X said. I started with the idea of a Nursing Home Journal and am being deflected into a study of one patient, the one always under my eye. I hardly get beyond passing the time of day with the others, partly because I am always walking in a straight line when I go out of the room, and when they stop at the door their conversation seems limited to "How are you?" or "Nice day." The men opposite both come over out of neighborliness, but one, Mr. H. (the 92-year-old) is deaf and what we have is an exchange of good will. He also pats and strokes Mrs. R. who retains her charm for men and responds to it; the other, who has had half his stomach removed and lives on a dreadful diet, including hot water, always comes over and says, "Well, it will soon be dinnertime," or "What will it be today, hamburger?" He is tall and kind and gentle and when he first came used to pace about and say, "This is a good place to die in," but now seems less restive. Communication is all with the nurses for most of us—the young, the fresh, with their sense of a long future.

Sometimes I wonder if it's fair to write, even for one pair of eyes, about Mrs. R. when she's in the room and blind. Sometimes too I dislike the writer's (in my case the unsuccessful writer's) notetaking attitude to experience. Mrs. R. at least is not exploiting anyone even in private. Her freedom from self-consciousness is part of her charm, when she is charming. I'll never forget her when the Singing Friars of St. Hyacinth's Seminary were here and we'd, as usual, cut their performance and she went out into the hall as they were coming out, still singing and playing their guitars, and came back to the room leading half a dozen young men by the hand, her face radiant. She said, "See what I've found?" She must have been beautiful and at times now I'd want to paint her, if I could paint—the red velvet dressing gown, the red ribbon in her hair, the eyes that don't look blind, the smile.

April 26

Reading Brendan Gill's *Here at the New Yorker*. There is an element of self-satisfaction in B.G. which prevents his ever becoming as great as the better men, often dislikable, like John O'Hara and Thurber, he writes of. But he's bright enough, witty enough to sum them up and big enough to admire their work. I think he hated Thurber, but there's something devastating in T's scrawling "Too late" over and over on the walls in his blind old age. B.G. knows a bit too about the way writers exploit their experience. (And I encouraged students to do just that.) And I am grateful to him for writing of E. B. White with love. Ross emerges for me throughout better than in Thurber's book. I think its reviews, the ones I've seen, have not been very fair to it.

I am not a bit interested in palindromes (he mentions the *N.Y.* writers who carried on an endless contest in them) but "Rats live on no evil star" is a nice one. No evil star, just "this little darke starre whereon we live." There is something in the narrow cells, the eccentricities and loneliness and even madness (the man who wound up toy trains in bars) that made the *New Yorker*. Did it take all the drink too? B.G. is something of a drink snob, quantitative not qualitative. But he is reporting facts. Mrs. R. has glowered all day. I tremble for what they'll do wrong, putting her to bed.

Thinking of the *New Yorker* and the quantities of alcohol —abstinence could not have created it, that kind. Yet there is a Puritan self-denial in the long hours of work, of checking and rechecking, getting things right. Maybe that happens on any good newspaper too, for facts, for grammar (not the Holyoke *Transcript-Telegram*) but perhaps not quite in the same way for tone. I wonder. Maybe *Playboy* insists on its own tone as earnestly as Ross or Shawn. The *T.T.* has no tone.

In the end: B. Gill made me laugh several times and heaven knows I'm grateful for that. What I miss is someone to read these paragraphs to—he isn't always such a lightweight as he likes to make himself sound.

I hear a shout "Man on the floor" again. I wonder that we never hear "Woman on the floor."

From the *New Yorker* itself, Michael Arlen on the sense of lost adventure in modern life and entertainment—the phrase "the relentless prosaic professionalism" of the astronauts. One might add "inarticulate." One couldn't bear to look at another moon landing (possibly Walter Cronkite could) but I was never moved, except by the pictures of the moon before they got there and of the earth after. The grotesque dress and the neat arrangements were a long way from the black ships. And the unwinged words!

April 29

In a way both days I wrote nothing down were high days. Sunday, I walked with the walker on the cement walk at the front in a strong, rather cold wind and felt as if I were climbing a mountain. The sun was in and out, the sky blue and grey, the clouds going by fast—an English day. But I wasn't thinking of anything but that I was walking in a wind and managed it.

Yesterday my moment of achievement came when I got out

of my chair without help—I haven't been able to repeat it. But oddly another high moment came when I was sitting under the hair dryer with Elizabeth and Millie, and drinking tea and looking out at the still bare trees against another grey-blue sky. It surprises me that it is possible to feel that kind of exhilaration when one is past seventy. Each time I feel it may be the last, but that is partly superstition, partly habit. Partly common sense.

Read the *New Republic* and the world returned. Having read T.R.B. and others on Vietnam, I read Frank Kermode on the perilous state of the arts in London—the taxes, the terrible prices, and the threat of extinction. As he says, no one wants the Old Vic to be turned into a Bingo hall.

Today the hired men are taking people for routine rides in wheelchairs. (It is possible they are volunteers, as any of them might be retirement age. One looks like a church deacon.) I think any way of getting out is good, but do not want that sort of professional jaunt. I walked my three cement blocks in the coolish sun.

April 30

Another exhausted day, with a visit to a Smith—and Johns Hopkins—graduate in the South Wing. I may be able to read to her sometimes as she can read only very large print. This gives me pleasure. I also got a brief walk in the air. After all of which, my mind is blank.

May 1

Began at breakfast with an unexpected May basket from the niece of the man opposite; she keeps his door decorated with seasonal symbols. I am glad she had removed the Easter bunnies and put up some rather charming parasols, not especially suitable for her uncle, who probably hasn't noticed the change anyway. Her May baskets are wide-open flowers—mine a crocus—with mints, etc., inside. It pleases me to see chubby little Mr. H. (roommate of Mr. O., the uncle) sitting at his table with a May basket, cutting up bread for the birds.

The other May 1st celebration was *The Marriage of Figaro* on *Morning Pro Musica.*
And now I'm going home.

May 4

Back from home, where one can talk about anything and read *Times* editorials aloud (Russell Baker on Kissinger "accompanied by sources close to Kissinger") and be with reading club again. Forsythia in magnificent bloom, hyacinths in the border, a show of all kinds of daffodils and narcissus. Only—only—am I going to be able to maintain myself here without killing Elizabeth? What can I do for Elizabeth?

A nurse has just come in with mercurochrome (or whatever is the latest equivalent) all over her elbow. "Oh, a patient scratched me," she said, quite lightly.

Toenails cut by a gentleman of the old school, with a flowing white moustache which seems to go back to the moustaches of my childhood, not to have anything to do with the younger ones with hair on the face. Something of the retired army man about him. Might bark, if angry.

May 5

Sudden fit of nostalgia for Maine, not brought on by reading Anne Lindbergh to Miss K. and her mention of a place at North Haven, but by a rambling plan, as I ate my supper, for Elizabeth's possible visit there this summer. No doubt North Haven began it, with the image of the hills of Islesboro seen from the Head of the Cape or perhaps Orr's Cove. But this was a violent desire for the meadow—I hope Phyllis Riley will never sell any of it off for building—and then the scramble down to the rocks, and the driftwood trees where one sat and looked out to islands. I remember crossing in a boat to pick blueberries on Van Black's "mountain" and saying to K. Wynd (who is dead), "I'd rather be here than anywhere else in the world." She said, "So would I." But we were only summer people, as I once tried to say in a poem. Maybe said.

This afternoon, Mrs. L., who once lived next door but has been moved to the West Wing, came down in her wheelchair, looking for her husband. (I have no idea how long he's been dead.) Last time she got herself over here, I heard her say, "I'm looking for a place to live. Somewhere nice and central." But when she did live over here she was surprised every night by her room, "Is that my room? Is that my bed?" She is both funny and admirable and I am sorry she left our corner. She is liked by all the staff and loved by Dick who finds it hard to bear that she is sometimes aware of her own confusion. No one cares for the lost and wandering more than Dick, who has something of the working priest, something of the doctor, but without solemnity—sometimes with high spirits. Something of the farmer too, of course, as he loves working on his small holding, with his pigs and bees. He is utterly different from Jimmy, younger of course, though both take pride in their work. Jimmy might think Dick a maverick. *His* attitude is more sergeant-majorly. Sometimes, coming on in a morning, he says, "Good morning, men" or biblically, "Good morning, people." Sometimes he says to a patient, "I don't want to hear another thing out of you." One can no more imagine Jimmy's putting his arms around an old woman whose head lolls as she makes inarticulate sounds, than Dick's saying, "Have yourself a shave, Mr. ———. It will make your bowels feel better."

May 6

And I hear it's 65°. My objective now is to get out in the sun. An hour or so of something near bliss listening to *Morning Pro Musica,* Bach "Jesu, meine freude." Dr. Arne (pleasant) and then the beginning of the celebration of Brahms' birthday, with the Academic Overture which never fails to excite me, as singing *Gaudeamus* did from the Scottish Students Songbook long ago.

Elsie's letter yesterday went on with the discussion of favorite flowers, which I started. She says she has to have fragrance, so her favorites are roses, sweet peas, rockets, mignonettes, and perhaps most of all freesias. Rocket I don't know and perhaps never shall. And freesias I have never seen growing out of doors so I didn't count them but I agree their scent is heavenly. I wonder if there were freesias among the clouds of fragrance in that Sicilian garden where I lost myself in pure sensuous delight, turning my back on the beastly, snobbish manager of the hotel and his contempt for me for not having luggage. (But that was an irrigated garden, one could hear water dropping from pipes all the while.)

May 7

Immediate passing spasm of dislike for Joan Fontaine's voice on the radio, advertising Arnold's cracked-wheat bread. Self-admiration, condescension, falsity, an intolerable forced half-laugh as she says, "Arnold's cracked-wheat bread is all it's cracked up to be."

I should record Mrs. R.'s going out for a wheelchair tour of grounds. She was just beginning to refuse when the nurse who asked her went on to say, "Here's a man all ready to take you." "A man?" said Mrs. R. and went with alacrity. I find these men are volunteers and I consider this a good kind of volunteer work, to be recommended to the hospitals, where one never gets one's nose outside.

I am charmed that Elizabeth Cragoe is having offers, as a result of her article, not only from literary agents but from people who want to send her wildflowers, even oxlips, which I never saw, and associate only with Titania.

May 8

It's getting too far into May, though here there isn't a leaf visible from my window, only flowers on one maple. There are, however, bluets in the grass as well as dandelions. I dare say E. Cragoe would like some bluets if only I could send her some. Visited by two of the Kings Daughters from the South Hadley church, who were here bringing over afghans—that is their volunteer work and a good many of these beds are gay with them—they were people I know from Hadley St., and Hadley St. is glorified in my eyes. I have stopped counting my visitors, as I want the list to end—not, of course, leaving me here. Long visit yesterday from Mary Jane Crocker, who brought back to mind a very nice but not spectacu-

841376

lar freshman class—in which Mary Jane brought her father to a discussion of Lear and he joined in, to my pleasure. She told me he died, at 52, of cancer.

May 12

Two orioles at once on a Japanese quince. But that was at home and not to be repeated. I think the orioles will not come close enough here. And never before have I been able to watch them for so long, the female first, hidden most of the time in the thickness of bloom—whatever color it is, pink, red, but I can't say what shade—the color of some roses, some camellias and a bird moving from branch to branch as I began to realize only orioles do. But it was ages before I saw her yellow breast and then the gorgeous male flew up and they both bounced—only that is too ungainly a word—from one branch to another or flew from one branch to another. Then for a moment another male arrived and I thought they were going to fight, while the female, unconcerned, went on pouncing on whatever she was getting from the bark, among the flowers. However I hanker for English primroses and cowslips, I have to admit this was an exotic sight I couldn't have had there. Meanwhile beside me, Serkin was playing the Waldstein. What was it I used to like so much in my very early days of poetry?—"A rainbow and a cuckoo, Lord / May never come again. May never come again / May never come / This side the tomb."

May 14

Life too much taken up with schemes—to get outside or being outside or having things done to me like washing, or hot packs or walking—to write the notes on nursing homes or the letters I ought to write. Shad bush in bloom, leaves still sparse, but coming. Sat on the walk outside, Meribeth on the one chair, Mary on her raincoat and my blanket, Irmina on paper bags, and the time passed imperceptibly like the movement of shadow on a dial.

May 15

A moment, while *Morning Pro Musica* was playing something dreary and Japanese, when I fell into the ditch where one contemplates the decay of the body all over again—and the cost of it. Mrs. Baker came in, bracing as ever, just off to Costa Rica where her son is, bearing a color TV set, a tent, and half a dozen other heavy bundles her son has asked her to take. (She drew the line at the new window for a Volkswagen) and cheered me up. When I said how much I wanted to get home and told her the obstacles, she said, "Go home. You'll be back with us, but go for as long as you can." I said I couldn't afford to come back. She said, "Sure you can. Go on Welfare like everybody else. *I* intend to go on Welfare when things break down. . . ." (Of course I contemplate the ignominy of Welfare when I'm in the ditch, as well as the loss of faculties.) I also think of the Cambodians, turned out of hospitals by the savage, single-minded Khmer Rouge.

Walking back to my room, I watched Bill N. stick his face out of the end door into the sun, but not his feet. He has sworn he won't go outside until he goes for good. He is sane, too, but angry with whomever it is who won't have him home.

Reading a review of Byron's letters and journals in the *New York Review*, in which lately I have found a bit to my taste. I was interested in the reviewer's comment, "The more private the writing of Byron, the more literary it becomes. The Journal contains passages with an extraordinary collage of quotations, fragments he shored against his ruins." It is almost inevitable if one has always read poetry. I feel as if my head is lined with it, but now all gaps and holes. In one entry B. asks, before his 26th birthday, "Is there anything in the future that can possibly console us for not being always *twenty-five?*" *That* I never thought—25 was all mixed up with the pains of learning to teach. Thirty, now—I remember being almost angry that someone suggested that I was 30 when I was 29.

Yesterday, reading the Mt. Holyoke program to the *Bacchae*, I felt the same pang I sometimes feel even yet for places not visited. And if I had known Greek, would I now be settling down with the *Bacchae?*

To go back to the article, which I have now finished and enjoyed, down to the discussion of dashes and de Selincourt's high moral tone with them. I looked back to find out if the reviewer Charles Rosen was indeed C.R. the pianist and he was. Let him review again.

May 16

Mixed, like the sun and shade when I sat out. Our conversation—Elizabeth appeared utterly unexpectedly—was checkered by the interruptions of various old men, all with good will—one who wears a religious medal and is nearly blind gave us strawberries and grapes last night. I think Elizabeth is afraid of having me home, and with reason, and that, in a way, our interrupted conversation on this (I refuse to say *dialogue*) is like the impasse my body has arrived at. I'd stay here till her book was finished if I could, but I am afraid that is much too long-term an affair for the insurance people. It isn't even any good resigning myself to staying here—one needs not only resignation but cash.

Rachel, who brings us our trays in the morning and gets me *Morning Pro Musica* as soon as she removes them, this morning brought me pheasant-eye narcissus and this afternoon came back in her time off to bring Mrs. R. flowers for her daughter leaving hospital. That is like Margaret, the nurse, taking her lunch hour to go home and get me trout to take home with me to South Hadley last Saturday. "Little nameless acts ———" P.S.: *unremembered* acts, but these won't be unremembered, I hope, for a long time.

Tonight, in spite of the fact that the *New Yorker* made me laugh several times, I feel a kind of desperation. I don't believe Elizabeth realizes that my ejection from here, when it comes, will be as sudden as from the hospital, but instead of saying, "You must go today," the insurance company will say six weeks later, "Your claims have been disallowed," after I've paid out vast sums.

Anne G. in her letter about her mother: "When I saw her coming with her beautiful 'Lady Anne' smile." That is good. I feel involved in all those family affections as well as the angers and recriminations.

May 18

Back from home again in summer weather, with everything —lilacs, dogwood, apple blossoms—rushing to its fall. Everything fragrant—I came back with viburnum, swamp azalea and lilies of the valley. I sat out in the midst of it and watched a wren considering our bird house. Today I heard it in full song as we sat at lunch by the open window. But even as Dick Remillard was measuring the steps for a ramp, I felt I'd never be back except as a visitor.

May 20

Knees bad, temperature outside good, orioles singing—yesterday I saw one and heard much birdsong in the woods I didn't recognize. Mrs. R. all dressed to go out and decorate the graves in Hadley, where she lived her life on the farm with her first husband —and hated it. I remember I used to feel "what a waste" at Arcadia as they carted off great armfuls of peonies for the graves. I felt they were robbing the garden for the dead. Now I feel it is good there are such pieties, which have lasted over the centuries and tie Antigone to unknown tribes and continents. (Similarly that's the kind of young life and energy that takes pleasure in knocking down gravestones. It isn't that I want a gravestone; I think of Jarvis Green scratching his father's name on a stone [now covered by the brambles and alder] and drawing a rough star. But I'd rather have it covered by brambles than overturned by crude life asserting itself in search of identity.)

I should record that Louise, the tough nurse, who nevertheless thought there was something to Mozart, returned last weekend and, though she threw things in every direction, picked up my *Little Treasury* and said to me, "Do you know the poem 'To thine own self be true?' "I said I knew the phrase. She went back and looked again and said "That's it—from *Hamlet* by William Shakespeare."

I realize I am falling down on my effort to record the nursing home life, as my time is so much taken up listening for orioles or writing letters or doing rough calculations on how I can either stay here or go home and not make Elizabeth suffer. I'd really like to sell her my half of the house for $1.00 now (that makes it legal). But the good daughters and a few good sons go on wheeling mothers and fathers up and down the halls, and people cry out, though no longer in this part of the wood.

I must note, however, that they have let one of the able-bodied patients—the gentle, quiet Mr. Wood who wheels his own wheelchair everywhere and sits down in it where he pleases—plant himself a garden. What I'm afraid of is that they'll spoil his vegetables in the cooking, but I think not many places would have the imagination and the land to let him do it at all.

Note—again after looking at *Country Life*—Bedlam hospital was a much handsomer building than this.

Hearing an appeal over TV for the Arthritis Society, I thought, "I won't leave my money to *them*." That is because they seem to me to get no further with all their research—they go on with the same palliatives and advice about rest and exercise without knowing a thing about how to arrest it or what causes it. I forgot too that I should not have any money to leave, though—perhaps it's common after 70—I still think of gladding this or that person's heart with a legacy or leaving money to a cause. Not a hospital which seems to me too much like the Pentagon in the inhuman price of its equipment for small legacies to matter. I liked the man I read of somewhere out west who'd left his money to an old folks' home in Sweden (Gol was the place, his native village) so that each patient could have a glass of wine every day. I don't know what I'd do for old people if I had the money, but see that they each had a teapot, certainly, and a more handsome kind of indestructible cup, a mohair blanket if I could afford it. But I suppose there are far too many who are beyond noticing such things and what can anyone do for them with money? Except for the money it takes to keep them in a place where they are kept clean and sometimes loved, though they may not notice even that.

Conversation overheard: nurse to a man (I don't know which), "Are you getting used to your new room now?" Patient, "The room's all right. I don't like *that* fellow though." Let us hope the fellow was not in the room. The roommate problem must be terribly hard on those who do the arranging as well as on many a patient. I wonder how Miss K. gets on with hers? When I go to see

Miss K. in the afternoon, the roommate looks as if she hated the sight of me.

May 23

Interested in some remarks on comedy in the *New Republic* —a review of *All in the Family*, of all things, a show I never found it possible to watch. "Comedy and death are old companions, as Yorick demonstrated, not merely in graveyard and funeral jokes but in substance. Both are forms of interruption. Both have social stature and command absolute attention. Neither is fully comprehensible to us in cause or meaning. Both are forms of criticism of reality, shattering pretense, showing people for what they are. To make a joke of something is to kill it. The terms of comedy are the terms of death: you're a riot, a scream, you break me up; you're killing me." But I feel I can't go along readily with all this and some of it I don't understand. The last sentence is specious—the terms might be other (in Yorkshire—"You're a caution, . . . you're a coughdrop"). I do not think death a criticism of reality, though it shows people for what they are—mortal. To make a joke of something is to kill it? I do not see that.

Paul A. comes shuffling down here every evening from the other end of the wing, where he lives. He is 96. He was once the janitor of the French church, I am told, and he feels he must still make the rounds of the building. Sometimes he comes several times and quite late, so that one often hears the nurses say, "Go home, Paul," and sometimes, "Marchez." Sometimes he stops and stares in, sometimes asks for a dollar. Sometimes he feels he has to go down cellar—there isn't one. He is always in short sleeves and braces and shuffling slippers that remind me of my grandfather's when I hear them.

May 26

Back from a weekend at home that was first sultry, then chilly. Most of the bloom gone already but for white lilac and heartsease and the lilies of the valley I brought back. Apart from the reading group, where we laughed, both at E. Bowen's seaside family and at each other's wit, it was a long interrupted conversation about the possible. We had to have it, but I have come back exhausted and depressed, feeling I am bound to wreck Elizabeth's life and her book if I go home. Meantime I make the house look less and less pleasing with the hall like a hospital bedroom which no one can escape if they come in at all. Something Puritan in me makes me feel I am taking the physical consequences of my sense of pride and ambition in my middle age. For two pins, I could howl. But we had to have this talk and, at length. . . . And now, maybe for a few days we should consider the lilies of the field.

May 27

They have as silly things told them in their staff meetings here as we had in some of our meetings—and I'm sure the orientation meetings for new members of the faculty were full of such silliness. I am told they spent an hour and a half in a meeting the other day in the course of which they were told to say, "Good morning, this is May 2nd. Next Monday will be Memorial Day." Amy, who cleans our room, gave a spirited demonstration of it this morning, adding, "The next meal will be lunch!" There is much badinage in the corridors that passes before I can record it, but which lightens life. Amy, Bert, the man who runs the vacuum cleaner—there are more.

Outside rather sultry before rain with the birds silent except for the ovenbird. The ovenbird is highly suitable for an old folks' home, though I took it he came of his own accord and was not placed here by the management as a symbol or a lesson in "what to make of a diminished thing."

The silliest song now on the radio is "A room without windows, a room without doors. / You and me, me and you / In a room without windows, etc." It suggests *The Pit and the Pendulum* or some kind of hell—No Exit. Paolo and Francesca.

May 31

Commencement and I shall see no one. A heavy grey day with a promise of thundershowers. My knees still ache from the ordeal of the hairdresser's chairs for an interminable time yesterday—

while the silver blonde, all flashing smile at times, did her monthly accounts and smoked. My feelings match Mrs. R.'s expression. Meanwhile the advertisements on the radio gave me spasms of disgust—all these bargains, all this enticement to borrow, and the weariness of the thought of the bank where your savings work harder than you do. To match the day, I put on my ugliest dress. To match my mood, I got one miserable cup of tea at lunch instead of a pot.

Sometimes I feel I fell with Richard Nixon—I'd just finished reading the Watergate transcripts in the *Times* when I fell on the hospital floor. There is no symbolism here, but I've never found the news as spellbinding since we got him out. But news isn't intended to be spellbinding.

June 1

Rain. Foggy and gloomy. I hope it clears for Commencement and they have Gettell's luck in Gettell's Folly.* I feel more than fifteen miles from it.

Found myself reading the ballads in the *Little Treasury*. How was anyone ever taken in by Chatterton? Surely phrases like "the storm increases" would have struck anyone who'd read real ballads, and the storm—I was reading "The Ballad of Chardee," which I'd never read before—has a strong flavor of Thomson's "Seasons." I can't remember whether Johnson was or was not taken in (and needn't) though I know he saw through Ossian.

But I soon got on to better things (passing by "Annabel Lee"). I still love "True Thomas," as I always did, though it was latish when I discovered it said art has magic in it and the tongue that cannot lie is the poet's. I love the argument True Thomas puts up against it. M.N.D. is about partly the same thing. "La Belle Dame" isn't. In the "Lady of Shalott," life smashed art all to pieces. I used to be haunted by the idea of the Lady of Shalott's breaking the rule, getting up and looking out and seeing nothing at all. Not as part of that poem, of course, but of another.

It occurs to me that, according to the evidence, the King and Queen of Elfland needed mortals as lovers, whereas Oberon and

* Amphitheater at Mount Holyoke College—Ed. note.

41

Titania didn't really—they played at it. This is not thought out and, I suspect, is not going to be.

"Edward" is like *Macbeth* in that retribution arrives from the first minute, though Edward accepted it from the first minute, while Macbeth hung on to his towers and his hall, and held off what he knew.

Overheard: Jimmy, "What's this about a bowel movement?" Patient, something not quite intelligible. Jimmy, "You want one?" P, "Yes." Jimmy, "You sound like I could find you one some place."

What is that quotation from the Bible—"Oh! my bowels, my bowels!" Something close to it. They are a great subject here, one way and another.

June 3

Rain (needed) and a bad light. Conversation overheard between two of the old men before I got up, before breakfast even. Bill N., who won't go out till he goes home. "There isn't a thing wrong with me. I'm not a bit better for being here. I could go any day only she won't have me." Mr. O., whose house is inhabited by a cat. "I feel your chances are better than mine. They told me I'd be here two weeks—that was last September." Home. Mr. N. so far revenges himself on circumstances that he won't even put clothes on. "They wouldn't have me," he said, "if I came and knocked the house down." Naturally I know nothing of their circumstances. All I know is that going home will be beset with difficulties, many I don't foresee. I hope it doesn't destroy anything. I don't want to knock the house down.

Strenuous interview with the chair man—the electrically operated chair, such as I use here, and which they are able to sell for a fancy price, being a monopoly. I do not want to and will not buy one till I see whether I can manage the other home conditions. Note at the same time—had just noted when he appeared—that Medex has paid nothing on my May bill. But the gloomy picture of conditions in the world in T.R.B. (sometime in the midst of this, Miss Cummings appeared and gave me the *New Republic*) raised my spirits. I heard a night nurse say last night as my roommate kept saying "Dear God," "I hear the name of God called on pretty often." I say thank God for people like T.R.B. and Anthony Lewis and Russell Baker and William Shawn. For the word, though I cannot go as far as the Word.

Another article on education by Ronald Berman interested me, especially on the matter of how Wittenberg has prepared Hamlet for life. "What earthly good would it have done Hamlet to study criminology at Wittenberg? Would that have prepared him for a country that was in fact a paradigm of the human mind? A country in which every lust including self-love and every sin including self-deceit was spelled out. . . . Life in a sense is what happens to you after you have faced necessity." As far as Hamlet was concerned, Wittenberg had perhaps given him the idea that he had to understand it before he could act in it. Or at least encouraged that idea which was in him. At worst, not killed it. Did it make Horatio knowledgeable about ghosts?

June 4

Low, because thanks to whatever, my knees feel as they have not felt since the day they cut off my aspirin on the theory of Dr. Brewster's young partner or assistant or whatever he is. I felt that whatever had taught me to recognize necessity has given me no power to cope with it. It seems to me life is a continual and probably endless series of facings of necessity, coping or failing to cope, not one looking in the face of things (except perhaps in a play). In reading poems, the recognition is accompanied by delight. In music I find more delight than recognition because I understand it less, or is it that the recognition is more generalized? One may weep without knowing why.

Mr. H. at 92 with one tooth is a self-appointed groundsman. He picks up sticks and breaks off rotten branches where he can. He gets a broom and sweeps up cigarette stubs. I have been told his passion for neatness in his room used to reduce one roommate he had to tears. And poor old Mr. G. who was in with him when I first came was a trial to him because he was incontinent. (I heard him give a plain-spoken account of this to his next—his present—chamber fellow, to whom I once heard him say, "You're the best I've had."

At this moment he is happy because he is listening to a ball game and the Red Sox are winning. Sometimes one hears him laugh aloud with joy at some master stroke.

Conversation between a father and daughter: Daughter, "What is it then? Are you discouraged?" F, "Yes." D, "You feel you're losing the battle?" F, "It's a losing battle." His tone a kind of unemphatic sadness.

June 7

Back after a mixed time at home. Now we have everything we can have to make life easy for me and all that's wrong is my knees. I never felt more unhopeful. *Wanhope*—that's what I feel. It isn't despair. The fact that it was wet all the time and we were shut up by damp green with only a few iris, a few peonies a long way off made it worse or was an expression of it. There was one moment, though, when the oriole came into full view on the lilac hedge and stayed a while after that, moving invisibly among the wet leaves. Of course there were good things, things a thousand miles from here like the reading group—we finished Elizabeth Bowen—and instead of beginning something else heard a spirited reading by Meribeth of V.'s review of all the Watergate books, full of literary allusions and footnotes. She said among other things that Richard Nixon was not like Oedipus. It was very hard to know what had been said or whether any of these books was to be recommended above another. Another good hour was hearing Buckley interview Helen Vlechos and two other Greeks, whose names I don't remember and who were both very intelligent and able—one is now a cabinet minister—but whose command of English was lesser than H.V.'s and so their wit less quick and flashing. Elizabeth and I got little conversation except on practical and immediate things, leaving me as usual with the feeling that I can't take all this from her, it's too hard on her body and mind. She told me she found plans for me coming into the forefront of her mind when she was working on her book. This matters to me more than anything.

Anyhow, back to the "yellow ribbon round the great oak tree" (Sherwood Forest or Boscobel) and "The Way We Were," the lamplighter apartments which have everything and Joan Fontaine's cultivated horrid praise of Arnold bread—and the same scraps of bad news between. And back to prefabricated turkey sliced off a roll, to instant mashed potatoes, peas and carrots out of cans, sweet puddings out of packages. And Mr. O. saying "Pretty near time to eat, I guess."

June 10

I want to copy Thomas's list of Yorkshire words he remembered into something a bit more permanent than a letter. This is his order.*

wishin—cushion
piggin—a lading can
ass-neuk—space under kitchen fire
sam t'asses—sweep up the ashes
cloise—field (I would add pay-cloise)
call(?)—appetite
cake or tommy—bread (I heard only new-cake)
nattercan—worrier (I heard natter-nangs)
mad higg—a fit of temper
guinge—earwig
mistal—cow byre
ganzie—blazer (I heard it for jersey—the jerseys of those
   days)
pobs—bread and milk
pike—spot on face, boil (sty on eye?) (Park?)
joy—term of endearment (also *doy*)
lop—flea
playing—out of work
laiking—playing
marlake—play about, mess about (I never heard)
cart on—play boisterously
pay—beat in a fight
think on—remember
side—tidy up
slart—spill (I heard *slout*)
sup—drink
bleg—blackberry (also verb: to go blegging)

* What follows is a sampling of the list—Ed. note.

shutter—rain heavily (shuttering *down*?)
lig—lie
threat—argue (to me *threat* suggests dominance in argument, e.g., he threated me down)
nont—aunt (cf. nuncle)
bide—bear
mash—pour boiling water on—*tea*
irkle—wrinkle
faint—smelly (but a certain kind of smell, not a stink. Dickens uses it.)
nantling—trivial
smittling—infectious
right set up—pleased (also *suited*)
maungy—peevish
middling—a lot
dowly—ill, poorly (sometimes badly)
meatwhole—able to enjoy food (I never heard)
throng—busy
ikey—haughty
nesh—sore (cf. M. English)
clemmed—hungry (cf. starved—cold)
brussen—bursting (brussen bubble)
fresh—worse for drink
stiff—fat
get agaate—get going
wick—lively (wick as an eel)
bray—beat
neck—swallow ("I could fair neck a pint")
champion—excellent (the ultimate in praise)
nigh on—nearly
face ache—toothache
winterhedge—clotheshorse (my favorite)
dateless—stupid
frame yourself—make an effort (I like this)
owered wi'—finished with
stalled—bored
onny rooad—anyway
ligger on—(cow between lactations)
living tally—cohabiting

46

car quaht—keep quiet
feel no rooad—feel ill
better ner like—better than expected (Mr. Bronte)
not but that—nevertheless
coit—coat ("It's warmer by a coit")
play bonny—behaving like a child
on't mending hand—getting better
pop his clogs—die
like used as indicative—did to see him, like? (But this is like
    the modern use among the inarticulate young except
    that "that" fills in every pause.)

I would like to add *fratch*—quarrel, which I like. Actually a number of Thomas's words I've not heard, especially the things that come out of his Farsley patients' vocabulary. One of the words I used to miss was *Nay*—not as a simple negative, but as a disapproving comment on a situation. "Nay, lass." Also *capped, faircapped.*

Having worked myself into a mood of semi-nostalgia about Yorkshire (where I don't want to live), I opened *Country Life* at a picture of a *prith stool* in Yorkshire in a village I'd never heard of, Sprotborough. Apparently there are prith stools in Yorkshire at Hexham (Northumberland?) and Beverly. It is a variant on the sanctuary knocker I'd never heard of and safer, somehow. I liked it. There was also a good picture of a packhorse bridge over Calva Beck in Cumberland, one of the oldest, with the information that the packhorse bridges had been built to take the place of mountain passes for the donkey trains, so perhaps an ancestor of my great-great-grandfather Wm. Clough who rode over packhorse bridges was struggling across the Honister or Winlatter or Kirkshire or something—my geography is vague—with his fleeces. One deprivation here is that one can look nothing up, but then I can't look up things at home without inconveniencing someone else. I haven't been able to lift a dictionary for years.

Meanwhile the bad news of the economy continues to come at intervals over the radio, and Mr. H. opposite, whom I observed earlier today with a broom is bragging, "There's one thing I can do. I can clean up. Ha! I'm a young man."

June 11

A morning so full of events that I am not dressed yet. A bath from which I was hardly dry when Dr. Brock came and the hot packs arrived before the doctor left. Meantime the nurse had to go to lunch.

Going back to yesterday. I feel there is a part of me that could have puttered away very happily at place names and dialect words, etc., if I'd been in the circumstances of an eighteenth-century country gentleman. So could Thomas have, of course—only he'd have managed his estates too, at least his "prospects" and temples or whatever he had. I'm not sure he'd have got enough chance at flower-growing. I think the Rev. William Cole was probably a happy man. I would not have wished to be an eighteenth-century woman. And if I'd had the money to choose language and puttering, I would not because I wanted Shakespeare and Milton and, though I did not know it then, Eliot, Yeats, and Wallace Stevens.

We cast a small die—I am to go home for a week.

June 12

The mother who complains and the daughter who pushed her wheelchair came to call on us last night. The mother confines her conversation to Mrs. R. as if I were not there. "Who's this then? (me) Do you find yourself comfortable with her?" The daughter and I laughed. The daughter then came over to talk to me and said, in what would have been an audible voice if the mother had not been so self-absorbed, "She has a sharp enough mind but uncultivated. She says things like that." The next thing she said to Mrs. R. was, "Who pays for you here?"

June 13

Reading a *Sunday Times Magazine* article on the widespread use of the *argumentium ad hominem* in academic institutions (in this case excluding speakers because of their associations), I thought that the Greeks (I am reading Thucydides by fits and starts) always tried reason—sometimes in the end they took to arms—and one's spirits are raised by the clearheadedness and often fairmindedness. (Of course with Melos it was the clearheadedness of *realpolitik*—the other side, Hitler and any one who if he doesn't get it will "take the thing he keeps.") Yesterday was discussing the Greek—and Viking—wars with Meribeth and Mary as compared with ours. The winter for withdrawal, mending the ships and perhaps a bit of reflection. There is no closed season on nuclear weapons.

I might record Mrs. R.'s silent tantrum when Dr. Brock was here. She obviously had enough control not to snap out or swear at the nurse who was washing her and who had done something wrong, but not enough to control her movements. She beat her feet against the foot of the bed like a child. I observed this through a chink in the curtain while the doctor sat with his back to her. And this is only an early stage of the unreason which may face one and which I dread, hopefully only at intervals, like real anarchy in the large world.

June 14

Notes on further research with popular songs. I've just heard one that begins, "How could I be so unsensitive?" a sentiment that never occurred in the popular songs of my day and ended with the icy *stare* he gave her—what else could he do when love was no longer *there*?* There is another in which the man packs his suitcase and slips down the stairs—it could never be the same again. And another in which he's late from the office again and she is going to mix—or fix—him a dry martini. There is another however which says why don't we pool our resources and join forces. And I just this moment misjudged one in which I was certain—because he was going to wake her up—that the something he had to say was that it wouldn't work, he had to leave her, etc., but no, what he had to say was "I love you," just as in the old days before they went to bed first.

One of the night nurses said to me—it was already light—apropos of my heartsease/johnny-jump-up, that she often found them where her grandmother had planted them. I said how rare to

* Misquoted—"What was I to do / but turn and stare in icy silence? / What else can one do / When a love affair is over?" Rather worse behavior on the whole.

live in a house where one's grandmother had planted things and she told me her children were the fifth generation to grow up in that house. That is a very rare kind of stability nowadays. But probably some of her children will take off with packs on their backs to Nepal or somewhere. Yet one of them may live to want the house—I hope so.

A low day, not desperate, but thick and lethargic. Nevertheless I heard wood thrushes outside.

June 15

Another low day, within and without. Broke off from reading Hannah Arendt on chaos invading the world, to walk on ruining knees, while up and down the hall people were yelling, "Nurse, Nurse," and a long way off Mrs. Sullivan was still calling "Martha." Mrs. R. has not yet her footstool or sheepskin. Mr. O. has lost his billfold and social security number. Clouds very low. If I come back after my week, I know very well what I come back to. But worse.

Teased by the passage I've read so often in *Paradise Lost* which I can't remember—"here length and breadth and depth and height are lost" (only that can't be right). In the microcosm I think its counterpart is no alphabet and no multiplication table along with the loss of personal law of all kinds till there is only the part of one that suffers and calls for help. This is like refugees on the road, except that some of the younger ones may have hope and live to realize it.

It seems as if the American Bicentennial can be celebrated only in fancy dress. (It is H. Arendt made me think of the bicentennial as her article is called "A Bicentennial Address"—the same theme as Jonathan Schell in the *New Yorker*. That is, image-making as policy. All very true and very depressing.)

Went to see Miss K. and say goodbye for a week. We somehow got on to what Faust sold his soul for and she said, "Nixon sold his soul for power." But, one feels, to a lesser devil than Mephistopheles, though the stakes were high enough. I wish I could think of the names of some of the smaller medieval devils. And yet for someone who wanted and got the crown. . . . One thing is sure, though, one can't make a tragedy out of him. The language is wrong. Perhaps one needs the lesser devils for the underlings. I thought we'd seen everything so far as Watergate is concerned, but Jonathan Schell has produced several new memos from Jeb Magruder to Haldeman—we haven't got to Colson yet. And there seems to have been no point at which any of them struck a bargain with any devil, or repented. No clock will strike midnight perhaps for any of them—or would they know?

June 18

Anniversary of my coming in. I sit all clean and exercised waiting to experiment with going home. Heavy, sunless weather of the kind we've had so much of. Impossible to read the omens.

June 25

Back. On the radio a man is singing, "Like a bridge over troubled water I will lay me down." I try to tell myself of all the people who are worse off than I am, and try not to feel impatient with the small things which through familiarity had half-endeared themselves. I should think of the pleasures of sitting out in the garden at home with the roses, the glimpse of an oriole or a cardinal and the cock crowing in the early morning, the conversations gone over the mill, Buckley and Clare Boothe Luce, fencing not exactly like Mirabell and Millamant but on the tradition of social comedy, food and wine, slides of Samarkand which made one want to read about the real Tamburlaine—and that V. has gone to an international conference in Mexico City for and about women and Jeb Magruder has got a job as vice president in charge of communications for a religious society called "Young Life."

". . . having to construct something on which to rejoice," only I can't say "Therefore I rejoice." Yet, if ever. Perhaps now as much as ever.

June 26

Committed myself to a picnic as a means of getting outside on a fine day. Found myself getting annoyed at the slapdash, clumsy unimaginative ways of a nurse, who is at least cheerful, quiet, and unruffled, and I thought that if I stayed here I could turn into an old crab easily enough. Good temper is a function of hope or of the sense of well-being, which must have hope in it unnoticed.

The picnic was no better and no worse than I thought. The air was good and the temperature just right. Conversation with Miss Z., former Smith faculty, was at least about people I knew. Food indifferent and without tea. The best thing was talking to Mrs. Maxwell between whiles and getting inspired—partly as a result of my bumpy ride out there in a metal bath chair with the seat cut out—to write to my congressman, Silvio Conte, telling him the county hospital in his district hadn't enough wheelchairs. I thought he might even know some minor philanthropists. At least this is a change from all the letters he'll get asking him to vote for this or that, to break Ford's veto or sustain it.

June 27

I noted that several of the ninety-year-olds enjoyed their food yesterday more than I did and could eat cucumbers and sauerkraut and onions and peppers better than I could. Not worth being 90 for, though, even if one acquired their appetites. Miss Z. next to me, who *is* 90 and has all her faculties, said she felt 90 was quite enough. One woman at the end of the table who did not eat made plaintive noises all the time, but she does the same thing even when her daughter is wheeling her in a wheelchair. Mrs. Sullivan at another table was still calling out "Martha," and once in a while someone would tell her, "Martha's at work, Kathleen." Miss Z. said, "Does one ever get used to these sounds?" I suppose the answer is yes and no. One cannot hear them for some time and then they sweep over one again, not a *memento mori* but a memento of how it is, not being able to die.

June 28

Low, but I can console myself and there are so many who can't—here, not to go outside these narrow boundaries. I can read Jonathan Schell and think how admirably he puts things together (and as an old pedagogue think what a good text it would have made for old-style freshman English or Exposition) without verbal fireworks, but with such admirable clarity and justness of perception, simplifying itself out into a sentence, now and then, which clinches something without being an epigram. One speculates again on hells and the Nixon men and I say, "I must read Dante again," almost knowing I won't. Patrick Buchanan should rank very low—upside down with the Pardoner? I wonder if either P.B. or Dean believed in the President? (Haldeman, I think, did, like poor Porter. Not Dean.) Did they just headily enjoy the unprecedented sensation of power and manipulation? When all the instructions had gone out, just about every spy, saboteur, conman, extortionist, faker, imposter, informer, burglar, mugger and bagman—for that astonishingly is what they were—in the employ of the White House was at work manufacturing the appearance of public support for the President. And Nixon was creating the impression of a man of peace. And Kissinger was being photographed smiling with people like Dobrynin. Surely there never was such a structure of wheels within wheels of appearances.

Heard a man in the corridor say, "Tomorrow I'm going to take a hearse." It's been that sort of day.

June 30

Yesterday, at home, was unclouded except in the sky. But I have the sensation of it all vanishing, of my not being able to get in the car or stand up at all, and I go back to the small sums of money which won't add up to the cost of staying where I don't want to be, "living and partially living."

July 1

Another note on popular songs—a theme I don't care for: "This is *my* life," "I'd still be me" and the brag of one who had taken highway and by-way but what is more, "I did it my way." Yet I have no doubt I felt that same self-assertiveness, though without consciously glorifying it, and made other people pay for it. I felt it when I ran away from my parents, felt it with a conviction that seemed like revelation when I gave up my job in Canada without having another. My leaving Texas, while less blind, was self-assertive, too, egotistical. I thought, "I can do better than this," but that's still, I suppose, "This is *my* life." I just don't like to hear these not very good tenors bawling it over the air.

Reading what seems to me a sound (though how do I know whether it's sound?) but not brilliant book by Desmond Seward on Henri Quatre. I don't like murders in high places one bit better than our murders in the streets (they had their murders in the streets too). But I am more terrified and horrified at competitions in nuclear weapons and the sale of nuclear weapons. I suppose it's Krupp and scrap iron to Germany all over again, but worse, more calculated and conscienceless.

Yesterday I demonstrated to myself that I was not going to be able to take it if I have to stay here; I refuse to say, "No way," which in any case by this time may be old-fashioned. Apart from song hits, I couldn't be less aware of fashions in anything.

This morning heard Mozart's Piano Concerto 24 and I am almost ready to say it is my favorite of all piano concertos—one of the earliest records we bought on the strength of a review, and a joy forever. At the time it led us to go and hear Paul Badura-Skoda in Springfield. He made one feel he could play Mozart all night.

July 3

There was much good in yesterday, including the fact that my knees worked better—better than today. I managed to get outside twice, mostly in the company of the old benchers. One who is 95 told me he'd lost his wife ten years ago after sixty-five years of marriage. "And when you lose your wife. . . ." he said and couldn't go on. I couldn't say much that he could hear. He wears a religious medal and, no doubt, waits upon the good Lord's time for him. I come nearest to conversation with Mr. O., who at least knows a bird when he sees one, and is always gentle and courteous, but he too is going deaf, as no doubt I shall go. Mr. H. went to mass for the first time since he came here. Mr. O. said, "Mister's gone to mass. I can't believe it. He's told the priest he didn't want to see him at all. He said, 'I know where I'm going!' " But he suddenly went. Out of doors, a perfect summer day.

Today another perfect summer day, when I felt for a short time what may be the height of bliss for a septuagenarian with crippled knees. The place was only just round the corner from here, in the shade with a wind blowing, among ferns, and on clover, with long grasses across the road blowing as I have always loved to see grasses blow, whether in a hayfield, cornfield, or on a walk as at the Malvern cottage. And of course in the meadow in Maine. I remember how my first summer in Maine was full of the sense of "days bound each to each," etc. Eating out of doors in the company one loves has been a constant pleasure in my life. Once there was talk on a ship—the old, slow, Baltimore Mail Line—of making the passengers get together and each tell the high moment of his summer vacation. Fortunately it never happened, but I remember telling the young woman I saw most of on that nice slow voyage that I thought mine was biting into a macaroon on Brighton beach—one of those many days of a long sunny summer when G. and S. lived at Brighton and we had sun, sea, tea (bought in a teapot in a little hut) so many times. The macaroon moment must have been an apotheosis. Like an adolescent I must say, "I have had this" and not, "I must pay for this." Or even, "I am paying."

July 6

I must have found nothing noteworthy on the 4th, as I remember nothing but a brief glance at Massachusetts on TV (Charles Kuralt) with tombstones of John Adams, Paul Revere, glimpses of the Old North Church, Old South Church, and the embattled bridge at Concord. Nicely put together. Part of the rest at least must have been spent in reading J. Schell on the horrors of the Republican convention 1972, every word written in the White House. We had a patriotic placemat.

Yesterday I was home and there were very good stretches, especially when we sat out in the evening to drink our coffee and a catbird came in the roses. But I felt terribly inadequate hearing two active (retired) colleagues so full of all their activities and overflowing with the life-force.

Today I saw what I took to be a new bird, as big as a flicker—pale fawn on head and breast. It clung to the wires a minute and was gone and I thought I'll never see it again, anymore than I ever saw a second yellow-hammer—after where?—somewhere near Wells, I think. Or a second hawk, close up, like the one in Maine who scolded us for being there. Now I wonder if it can have been an immature flicker without its markings—it had a ragged look, like young birds not long out of the nest.

Grateful for an article on night by Barry Lopez *(Audubon)* which made me realize it was a long time since I'd seen night skies as clear as those at Cape Rosier and brought back the marvelous, cold night when we stepped outside the house and saw the Northern Lights. Auroras of Autumn.

July 7

The day of the scarlet tanager. The picnic place was the same, with Elizabeth and Joan instead of Elizabeth and A.J. but the same sense of having nothing else to wish for, when the scarlet tanager (my second all my life) paused for a moment for us to see him, then flew across. (Joan I am sure felt there were other things to wish for and Elizabeth no doubt after a while wanted to get back to her book.) I sound as gushing as Anne Morrow Lindbergh in her freshman year.

Violent quarrel audible between two men a room away. One (95 and nearly blind, though tall and upright) is calling the other a "God damned stinking Polock." Actually both are "Polocks" and both speak Polish.* The other one has muscular dystrophy and the painful speech of one who was born deaf and dumb. The big one, who is angry, is imitating the uncouth sounds the other makes—I don't know how the nurses understand him, but they do. It is horrible. The tall man is the one who always wears the religious medal and who to us is very polite, calling us "Young ladies"—but he can't see. I wonder how long one hangs on to the amenities?

July 8

I don't want a picture of the scarlet tanager on a bough of plum blossom—I feel rather that he gave definition to something, a boundary line to an hour of happiness.

* (I later heard the big one was Lithuanian.)

Scarlet, crossing from tree to tree
You gave line
To an hour of happiness.

That, I am sure, is a wrong arrangement of syllables and I never cared for the haiku, never read a simple one that took my breath away. I can't see any possible way I can get the sweet fern and crushed sassafras into it.

On the amenities, again minor irritations over having my dirty stockings left on the table, not exactly for lunch but at lunchtime, and at other minor failures of imagination in the same slow, bull-in-a-china-shop nurse, made me aware how easy it would be to cross the line. Elizabeth says one doesn't call people stinkers or bitches without some previous habit of it. I don't know.

Another advertisement over the radio I dislike. The product is Tab, which is, I think, a drink; the theme song is "Be good to yourself" and the instrument a girl who's going to paint her toenails, drink Tab and be good to herself. She irritates me in quite a different way from Joan Fontaine, descending and condescending to advertise bread.

July 10

There is absolutely no mystery in a hospital as an environment and institution. Any mystery is in the minds, perhaps the bodies also, of the people in it. Like a liner in the old days with its swept planks, meal gongs, and "activities." (Here a voice announces, "Activities are now over. Will you please return your patients.") Only in the liner the sea swept up to one's feet almost, broke on one's windows. Here the woods are across the road, cut back and sprayed (yet still full of birds and the hidden possibility of a fox or a deer). Just now I heard a cardinal as I stepped laboriously, with my walker, over the doorsill. I was struck by the fact that it delighted me, but meant little to the nice girl who was with me. She is going to be married. When I was a good deal older than she is, staying at Juniper Lodge in N.H., I remember wondering at the older people there who got so excited about a hermit thrush.

Mr. H. who has been clearing the grass of stones and came in in a muck of sweat is again exulting over his frail roommate. "I've been working see? You never do nothing." But he was very kind and gentle to Mrs. R., who is feeling ill, patting her hand and saying, "You take care of yourself, kid."

July 11

Suffered in the hairdresser's chair again, but not for as long as last time. Am in the last installment of Jonathan Schell, which has lost the diabolical fascination of Watergate but raises the hair by quotations from Kissinger on the strategy of limited war. He says "it may be necessary to face Armageddon." But one would have thought the facing of it would be enough to make a man so intelligent realize one can't monkey about with "limited war." I feel *his* hair should rise on end too "like squills upon the fretful porpentine." So should Ford's and Schlesinger's talking about "not ruling out the possibility." Would I rather be killed by a nuclear weapon than live to be 90? Yes, on personal grounds. No, emphatically because there are no personal grounds with nuclear weapons. It is the impersonality of Kissinger that so horrifies.

Another difficult attempt at conversation with Mr. W. of the religious medals. We were the only occupants of our rampart. He told me again about his wife and again, as Abram Armitage used to say, he "filled." He said, "Have you a husband living?" I said I never had one. He said, "God bless you." I had a real inclination to say, "I never had no husband."

One of the nurses, hearing of my letter to my congressman about wheelchairs, said, "You can write to him next time about commodes."

July 12

Dull, muggy, overcast. Sitting out a limited pleasure. Have just heard, at supper, a somewhat emotional account of the death of Ruffian, the race horse, which went to the length, rare on TV, of quoting a bit of the Book of Job on the horse, and I thought I must go back and read that whole thing and then thought of Chaucer on the horse "so horsely." I am sure Ruffian was horsely. And then, tangentially, of the Dauphin's horse in *Henry V*—a horse of another color (nutmeg?) but still. . . . Joan should make a collection of horse passages. Good letter from Susan.

July 14

My birthday yesterday was mixed, while last year's under the tree with champagne and cool shade on a true summer day, was unadulterated, though at that time I couldn't walk a step and sat in what they call a geri-chair—with a tray as in a child's high chair, for second childishness. Yesterday's was mixed because I have just about lost hope, though I have times when I forget I've lost it, clouded by rain, and by hangover symptoms of the cold that has lodged itself in this corner, laying some people very low. But there were so many good things, including a brief reading group meeting and the first chapter of *Howards End*. (I'd forgotten it was funny) and a good buffet supper with our last roast beef from the freezer—never to be replaced—and Paul's beans and Mary's rolls. And much talk. I don't think Joan is as thrilled with the idea of collecting passages on horses as anyone who can handle them so easily—and was an English major—should be. I immediately thought of the *Venus and Adonis* passage too, as well as the horses of Achilles. In prose my memory does not serve me so well. (N.B. The Green Knight of course and Gringolet.)

Wonderful letters today and the surprise of an extra birthday cake—and a hairbrush!—from the nurses, who came in a body, with Jimmy, too. I know they have the custom of doing this, but I thought I'd missed it by going home. I felt really touched, as I did by Nora's getting up at six to get me good roses for yesterday and bringing them out, though it was her vacation—and by Thomas's letter, which gave me a suffusion of family feeling and memories of the chimes at midnight.

Heavy rain, with flash-flood warnings and the windows at times blotted out. Have just heard an astronaut say that he thought the meeting with Russians in space, learning each other's language, etc., held out immense possibilities for cooperation *in space*. It may be that's the only place we'll achieve cooperation. (I think of Ralph Nader and the oilman—arguing or more than that on TV yesterday.) Detente out in the Milky Way. (I heard over the radio this morning that France was displaying some part of its latest nuclear weapon in the Bastille Day parade in Paris.)

I just remembered "At ilka teet o' her horse's main / Hung fifty silken bells and nine." Who's making this anthology, Joan or me?

July 15

There is Rosinante, of course, and D. H. Lawrence—end of *The Rainbow*. Are the horses described in Malory? So little is. Spenser must be full of horses—the one I especially remember, besides the Red Cross Knight's, is the one fleeing "like Pegasus his foal."

Heard the woman in charge of the dinner wagon talking about ways and means and the price of food and also the difficulty of knowing how much to cook, now that the staff, in protest against the higher prices they are charged for meals, have, most of them, taken to bringing their own lunch, but on wet days like this want to eat in the dining room. She mentioned one woman who works in the kitchen, for a pittance I am sure, who is supporting her family. I think too of all the nurses whose husbands are not working. One of them brought me tea, for my birthday, and a Chelsea bun at breakfast with a candle on it. I wonder at the way they never fail—or almost never—in cheerfulness.

Heard from my usual source, radio station WFCR, that Ravel had wanted *L'Après-midi d'un Faune* played at his funeral. I wonder if it was. It would not be my choice, but I don't want a funeral. Sometimes, narcissistically, I play with the idea of what passages I'd have read at a memorial service in Abbey Chapel in which not a word would be said about me. But I break down over the number. I remember being asked to choose the passages for Mrs. Stewart's memorial service and the fact that Henry Stahr who read them threw out, "We must endure our going hence, etc." I suppose it offended his ministerial soul.

July 16

Mr. W. of the medal has evidently been given Mr. D. as a roommate to take the place of the "stinking Polock" who has been taken to the hospital. I heard him welcome him warmly,

"You a good boy." (Mr. D., the kindly barber, is, I think, a good boy. I have never heard him complain, as he shoves himself about in his wheelchair. I find his speech hard to understand, and very limited, however.) Now big Mr. W. is telling him that when you lose your wife, you've lost everything, to which Mr. D. said, "I've lost everything, too," unemphatically, as if stating a fact.

Wonderful story in James Merrill's review of Cavafy—full of sentences I want to copy down—about a Greek mother telling her child to tell its bad dream to the electric light bulb, just as Clytemnestra told hers to the sun.

I am glad to have known James Merrill, however superficially. And of course deeply grateful for our semester of Auden, and the ride from Hartford with Wallace Stevens.

I can't copy all the things I'd like to in J.M.'s article, *NY Review of Books*, July 17, 1975 (strange how the *NYR* veers from the inbred and bleakly inferior, to something splendid one wouldn't have missed), but *will* copy one poem translated by Edmund Keeney and Philip Sherrard:

THE GOD ABANDONS ANTHONY

At midnight when you suddenly hear
an invisible procession going by
with exquisite music, voices,
don't mourn your luck that's failing now,
work gone wrong, your plans
all proving deceptive—don't mourn them uselessly:
as one long prepared and full of courage,
say goodbye to her, to Alexandria who is leaving.
Above all, don't fool yourself, don't say
it was a dream, your ears deceived you:
don't degrade yourself with empty hopes like these.
As one long prepared, and full of courage,
as is right for you who were given this kind of city,
go firmly to the window
and listen with deep emotion,
but not with whining, the pleas of a coward;
listen—your final pleasure—to the voices,
to the exquisite music of that strange procession,
and say goodbye to her, to the Alexandria you are losing.

July 17

A picnic, but this time we were caught in a thundershower, in which nevertheless there was a certain exhilaration. Joan held the *New York Times* up as a screen and we had the trees.

Last night, awake for a short time I heard someone crying over and over, "Get me out," then, "Man, get me out," then, "People, get me out." I went back to sleep to it.

Am interested, reading K. Clark's autobiography, in the way he found his vocation suddenly and in spite of everything he'd been brought up with in his shooting, fishing, philistine surroundings. (Also, briefly, in the fact that he was born on the same day I was.) I think he is honest on his own kind of gift and kind of mind. I feel I owe him a good deal for *Landscape into Art* and his book on the nude. Whether he is a scholar or not; more than so many scholars.

July 19

Yesterday so low a day—except for a visit from Joan—physically and mentally that I felt, looking across at Mrs. R. holding compresses to her eye and feeling many degrees lower than I was, that I could easily sink into that kind of hopeless fatalism and in less time than the five years more of living she has had. Today at least I could pay a bill (the lowest rung yet on the ladder of pulling oneself out), finish a letter, and contemplate another. But I saw my next-door neighbor go home with deep envy.

July 21

Back after a night at home I had not planned for, but yesterday the heavens opened and after several hours of it, I decided to stay, thankful that I could. But nights are all I can look forward to. Then, not even nights. It is as if "Time is, Time was, Time is past" has happened almost as fast as with Friar Bacon's head. I felt Mrs. R.'s depression and physical distress settle on me as soon as I got in the room and couldn't for a while dispel it even for myself. As for driving the clouds away from her, I'm lacking in the energy and the love—and perhaps the love that lifts other people out of the ditch depends a bit on energy. So I made excuses for myself, unlike the saints.

July 22

Last night had a very interesting conversation with Dick, who had a kind of change of heart suddenly, while his army column or whatever the word is was held up by some stoppage —I won't say a traffic light. Having gone from private to captain in seven years, he saw his future in a flash and saw he had to get out. So now he works for next to nothing, grows his own food, reads late at night, and is a happy man. He also goes to Quaker meetings.

Read in *NYT* large print edition (Miss K.'s) that Richard Nixon had been photographed with bare feet. This gave me a shock, as if I'd assumed his clothes didn't come off. He was, however, wearing a dark jacket with the presidential seal, even on the beach. Utterly revolting.

July 23

Another picnic, but without a scarlet tanager. Not that I expect one—that is Nature, whereas in art one can go back and look again, if one has the legs, the eyes, the money. I recovered something of my feeling for Sicily—is it twenty-two years ago?—talking to Ruth L. about her visit there this summer. Only I can't summon up the feeling of looking at the Copella Palatine or Monreale —I remember looking at the flowers under a grey sky at Monreale, and the Arab fountain—also the man and woman who got on the street car to entertain us and took a collection—could it be that she sang and he played an accordion? And hearing how Ruth was robbed by boys in the street and went charging up to the slum houses where she saw them disappear—I had a vivid memory of little boys pursuing me down a dubious narrow street to the sea, with courts full of wet sheets—the always damp sheets one encountered on the beds. But little boys didn't snatch handbags in those days. As I think of it, none of the memories of mosaics and capitals are like the old men at Enna in their long black cloaks, or the garden of the San Domenico, where I could turn my back on the black beetle of a manager or the feeling of being lost in the quarry garden at Siracusa. It was something of being alone in a really strange country and surviving. It is as if I recalled how it was at the theater in Siracusa in the early morning *because* of the two donkeys braying at one another and refusing to give ground.*

Mrs. R., who has been to the eye doctor, has just been told that one eye is deteriorating so rapidly that she'll have no sight at all. She is worn, her hand can hardly hold up her head. The big man across the way goes on talking in a booming voice. Mr. D., his roommate, says, "Yesh." Every night the big man thanks God and the Lord Jesus Christ for his good supper.

July 24

Poem in the *New Yorker* by Galway Kinnell which I don't think good but the argument of which interests me—I don't know how old he is because I missed, deliberately, his reading of his poems at Mt. H. His thesis is "Wait. . . . Personal events will become interesting again," which they will. But when he says, "Be there to hear it it will be the only time" (so far, so good)

Most of all to hear
The flute of your whole existence,
Rehearsed by the sorrows, play itself into total exhaustion,

I must object, in these surroundings. The total exhaustion silences the flute (I look at my roommate) and may be prolonged beyond hearing, one thinks now because one can still hear—if not resignedly. What one dreads is that the flute should stop years before the end of breath. Even Dick, who learns so much from patients who will never walk, never straighten out an arm or leg, never see, has to admit there is nothing for the vegetable state when one can't die. I would like an agreement, signed and sealed, that if I become so, no one will expose me at picnics, in the Happy

---

* I also have vivid sensations still of the train stopping at Roccapalumba—and getting out and eating a salami sandwich I bought on the platform, and then as the train went on, pulling itself out slowly, seeing and hearing a shepherd boy playing on a pipe. (I never saw that in Greece though I once heard shepherds singing as they drove the flocks home at Hadrian's Villa.) R.L. was too late, though she escaped the damp sheets, to hear a shepherd boy and a pastoral. Also she went CIAT.

Room or in any public place. Doesn't Lancelot Andrews have his bones exposed on his tomb in Winchester Cathedral? But those dead bones, though I don't like the ostentation of that kind of tomb, are at least over.

A review of Joseph Campbell's *The Masks of God* in the *New Yorker* (July 21) makes me feel I'd like to see the book to look at the pictures. (I remember J.C.'s lecture at Mt. H. and that I was not thrilled, thought it a little too much of a conjuring trick.) But I don't think Winthrop Sargent was the person to review it. (He says, for instance, that his illustrations "represent art not as aesthetics or realism, but as symbol or dream," as if anyone thought art aesthetics or thought realism anything but one kind of art.) When he says that if the book does not convince the reader that "Jung's hypothesis about the universal unconscious is correct," that reader is of the limited class of realists. But I do not see the need to postulate a *collective* unconsciousness—Jung always lost me there. Why must it be collective to account for the similarity of divine images? I feel as I do with the struggle when it's in the cosmos and not in man. Not that I want to deny the place of dream in art, but I won't say art is dream. Think of all the study of anatomy behind, say, the Sistine ceiling. This is so obvious that it isn't worth saying. The *New Yorker* should have done better. I'd like to talk about it to somebody.

July 25

I suppose the reason for the endless repetition of the talk here is that we lack subjects. Our health, the food. From across the hall comes assurance of the latest score of the Red Sox. People ask one another how many children they have, but by this time we know. All is personal and present. Only with the nurses do we get any variety and that is limited to clothes, houses, dogs, cats, vacations, once in a while old buildings, or Morgan horses. A few books. And I must thank the Rev. Mr. Montgomery for the variations in his prayers. (His ties, too, sometimes cheer me up.) And sometimes we talk in a limited way about music, mainly popular. (I am limited on music in any case and on popular music very much so.) I felt unreasonably pleased, though not very adequate, when Miss

K. came all the way from the South Wing to ask me what it was that was found in a croquet-ball box.

Jimmy has just remarked that he'll be retiring in twelve more years and added, "I'll never make it." Whereas what we are afraid of is that we may last twelve more years, still asking, "How are you *today*?" Then probably not caring how anyone else is today or any time.

One keeps on coming up against the fact that Ford has no brains, or vision, for want of which, etc.

July 26

Another note on the *me* theme in songs. "You've got to love me for what I am / For simply being me." I am afraid I've missed putting down a number of the other ones, where one of the parties concerned steps down the stairs in the early morning, but there are several. Nothing else worth recording except that it's a perfect summer day, after much 90° humidity.

July 28

Today I feel I can't see any possible way of staying here and keeping myself civilized. Last summer and all last winter I lived on hope, eating synthetic meat whose taste was sawdust because it was going to sustain me on the parallel bars (there were weeks those parallel bars were the crown of the day). At these moments, I am always visited by the knowledge that every one in my old life will find they get on very well without me. Then I descend and think if I had decent food, I'd have the excess of energy one needs to make people interested in seeing one. I don't want to be visited as a good work.

Another song on the radio that annoys me—they lifted "the forests of the night" (the man wants to be near her in the forests of the night) and then in the next line—I can't quote, which is just as well—he wants to stand by her when she blows out the candles on her cake.

An interesting review in the *Atlantic* of various books (Bradlee on Kennedy, Safire on Nixon, T. H. White on Nixon) called "Politics and Class" and the class element is interesting and perhaps especially so in Kennedy who said Nixon was "no class," as N. too obviously knew, but K. was conscious of not being a Bouvier. J.F.K. does not come out at all well in the reviews and bits of Bradlee's book I've read, but the anecdote of his getting angry over being given a silver-*plated* bowl by a governor is surprising. Of R.N., the reviewer (Richard Todd) said, "Neither White nor anyone else has persuaded me that Nixon ever said an interesting thing—ever revealed an individual taste, a moral sense, a psychological acuity that one could learn from. And yet he *is* a profoundly interesting man." Yes, but I still would not follow him further when he goes on to say he is tragic, though the comparison with *An American Tragedy* at least doesn't take him out of his depth as far as language goes. But I don't think he has the awareness even now for a tragic figure. I think he thinks he had bad luck. But how should I know?

This afternoon when I was sitting outside, the daughter of the big Lithuanian, who comes every day and plays rummy with him as if it were what she most wanted to do, said on her way in that she wanted to live to be 100 because she so much wanted to see how things would turn out. I hear she has a sick husband too. She made me think of the soldier in *Anthony and Cleopatra* who says, "Here's a gash like a T—here's one like an H" (or whatever he said). She filled me with shame, but even that didn't stop me feeling sorry for myself.

Heard the first mention of a sleeping pill in song.

President Ford took his first sauna bath and after beating himself with a birch (birch what?) pronounced it a delightful experience.

July 29

Another picnic, this time with Elizabeth, Joan, and Irmina, who provided interesting sidelights on the *Gazette* and who is always a pleasure to be with for her modesty and gentleness and humor. I admire her courage, along with her scholarliness. No birds and this time a few mosquitoes, but a perfect summer day and the distant echoes of the musical entertainment I'd missed only made it better.

July 30 (or 31—I think I've got a day out in my calendar)

I keep on being struck by the fact that the people who wait on us are working for very little. They grumble, but also laugh, as they push their mops and cleaners around in the corridor. They have children whose teeth have to be corrected, and things stolen and this or that expense for the car. Often with the women, their husbands are unemployed or part-time. Others, since the governor's threat of laying off state employees, go in fear for their wives or husbands. This is the Middle America Nixon used to talk about and which he (only now it's Ford) is gradually strangling. They are the ones—except for those already unemployed—who take it first. Elizabeth and I will be caught in it a little later, most of our friends later still. After all, I was young when I worked for next to nothing in the Depression and even so I still went home—once I came back with 75 cents in my pocket. It is the middle-aged ones here I feel most sorry for, old enough to be tired, young enough to have children who still depend on them, though I am sorry for the young nurses too whose husbands have been to college and can't get jobs and the humiliation of dependence, not just because they're men.

Visited Miss K., whose birthday it turned out to be and I think it was good for both. We had a subject—Nixon in the *Atlantic* book review—but got ourselves in round the edges. She is almost certain she is losing the sight of the second eye. This was followed by a wonderful surprise visit from Elizabeth and the complete relaxation of being at home with someone who knows all about one, as deep as one goes.

August 1

Took communion for the first time in my life, not from any real change of heart, but from my admiration of and liking for the Rev. Mr. Montgomery. I can't feel I was violating anything. If I'd stayed in Dallas I might have been confirmed because of Dean Moore. I might, but that would have meant a kind of perjury and I think I'd have stopped short of it.

Pleasure of having the Yorkshire nurse, who normally works in another wing. I asked her if she'd heard a few expressions on my list (she's probably 30) and she'd heard *capped* and *fratch* but not *throng*. She reminded me of *Na'then* (strong admonition) and said her husband had been laughed at for calling his lunch-box his *jock-box* when he first came over. I'd forgotten that use of *jock*. Apparently here it is indecent slang.

I asked Nancy when Mr. Drake takes his vacation. She said, "Never." This I believe. He can't trust the mice not to play.

Overheard the big Lithuanian say to Mr. H., "Get out of here you goddammed little Frenchman." What about I don't know, unless Mr. H. has been telling him where to throw his cigarette butts. He must be a very difficult man to room with. Only a man as meek and gentle as Mr. D. could please him. Yet no one is more free with blessings in the name of the Lord.

August 3

Home yesterday in spite of 100° heat. The heat in the afternoon was as bad as anything I remember, and yet it seemed as if one sweated out one's self-pity. I wasn't aware of anything but feeling hot. Really enjoyed another brief go at *Howards End*, the supper, and the talk, and *Agronsky and Company,* to say nothing of my friends.

Unsatisfactory reply, though courteous, from Conte, who says why don't I write to the local paper about wheelchairs. The answer is I do not wish to make an enemy of Mr. Drake, who, I am sure, likes the local publicity to take the form of pictures of people cutting birthday cakes or working earnestly at crafts.

Looking up an address in what I now use as an address book, I noted the many references to Donne's sermons scattered through and thought with a kind of dismay, like a sudden weight, of all the notes I'd taken in my life. Piles of them on Donne's sermons alone, never pushed into any kind of shape. But even if I'd got into *PMLA* what good would it have done me now? A stupid thing to say, and against all I believe and live by.

One constant thing in my long (already) stay here: "Tie a yellow ribbon on the great oak tree." They were singing it in June 1974; they are singing it now, this minute. I shall outlast it.

August 5

Yesterday was all my visit to the dentist. Fears, beforehand, after all this time that our dear Vassar Higgins was going to find a hundred cavities and shake his head, but instead he found only two little ones. I didn't exactly enjoy his excavation of tartar but I was much relieved. I had felt they were rotting away. Brief glimpse of Holyoke in my ride round the block in a wheelchair, as ugly as ever. I felt it was like the dream cities I sometimes walk in, except that I always dream of them as dark, with very little light from the unknown buildings, which aren't the place I'm looking for. I don't want to see Holyoke again, except that I hope I can be hauled to Vassar Higgins at need.

The return of Jimmy from his vacation means more badinage in the corridor again. I was glad to hear his voice.

Limited conversation outside, in the too great heat, with the Lithuanian. Much of it I missed but at one point he said, "Yes. When I am young man I was strong. I said to my son-in-law, 'You go down' because his knees was shaking. I said 'I climb the tree,' and I picked the apples." I have probably got in too many prepositions and conjunctions. It left the impression of a picture in a child's book, simple line and color. He added, "But I'm no good now." I can't think of a single thing to say to him that I can make him hear.

One present line of tea bags carries wise saws on the labels. Mine says, "Every force of nature has a double edge—water quenches thirst yet you can drown in it." But is that a double edge? Mrs. R.'s says, "Solitude is not the same as loneliness." Agreed.

A song now playing has just rhymed *you* with *gin and vermouth*.

August 7

Words leave like orioles in August. You saw them yesterday. What comes is a sparrow. The best left long ago like the cock pheasants in the glory of their Chinese rings when they marched up the border, hens following demurely (in a flurry of leaves). (There was one day the pheasants came in the snow and all the

while an enormous rabbit sat under a pine, still, with the pheas-
ants heading for something.) But perhaps I never had a word like
a cock pheasant—("Who has made a great peacock"). Still, better
the sparrows certain, that after all come alone, and the chance of a
bluejay with his great squawk (of self-assertion)—this is one—
than the fall sky, full of grackles all going. I don't mean death.*
Passing Mr. W.'s room, I heard him singing in Lithuanian. It
sounded like a folk song. The nurse and I stopped to listen. He was
lying on his bed and alone.

Reading the *Mt. H. Quarterly* was moved by the tribute to
Jo, not only for the truth of all they said about excitement over
learning and literature, but for Andrea's self-effacement in the
handling of it, calling in other students' opinions and quoting
them at length and yet putting her own stamp on it.

August 8

Still raining with a Noah's flood steadiness and promise of
keeping on. Very dark. Heard over the radio that Gerald Ford has
rounded out a year in office. It must be fact. Last night the feud—
if that is what it is—between Mr. W. and Mr. H. became a school-
boy water fight. When Mr. H. went to return the evening paper to
Mr. D., Mr. W. not only started yelling at him to get out, but
threw water over him, whereupon the goddam little Frenchman
went back quite deliberately to his room and got a glass of water
and threw it over Mr. W., who shouted in outrage. Several nurses
had to go in to calm him. All Mr. H. said was, "I got even with
him"; he didn't need any calming down. Well, they are both in
their nineties. I tried to think what institution of learning that I'd
been connected with had an annual water fight and decided it
must have been Hood.

August 9

I'd like to write a poem on these two old men, full of physical
force in their nineties and scrapping like boys. Mr. W. in particular has something of the terrible strength of an Old Testament fig-

---

* Drafts of poems in process are set in italics. For final version of this poem see
August 11, 1975 entry—Ed. note.

ure (I won't say *prophet* because I think his power is physical, the sheer "I'm alive" that we could do with more of in this room—though heaven knows I don't want to room with anyone of that degree of dominance. I feel Mr. D. has little room to breathe). What Scandinavian novel that I read in my youth had a hero who was always called a great barge of a man? (Jo calls all those novels *The Great Hunger* with the g—I've lost the term, *unvoiced?*—as in German.) There was a tremendous hullabaloo last night in the old man's room, not another quarrel with Mr. H. I think, but what sounded like an expression of outrage that such a person should come in his room, and a woman's voice (his daughter's?) telling him the room belonged to two people. But I'm sure he was a man to be afraid of in his youth, a man who'd fell you at a blow. Yet his daughters seem devoted to him. He is like an old tree of great height and girth, still standing.

The Rev. Mr. Montgomery had a beautiful shirt and tie yesterday. It pleases me that he is a dandy (or whatever is the modern term for dandy) without, I am sure, violating any ministerial conventions. A "good man," whose very minor vanity gives other people pleasure. I detest the Simeon Stylites type.

August 11

Yesterday at home was sad because of Edward's dangerous illness, which seemed like the further invasion of the dark into all our lives. "What we can expect," we said. And Joan *capable du tout* is leaving this week. I had the feeling that the next time I see her I may not be able to get in and out of a car. But I enjoyed a bit more of *Howards End*—I always forget E.M.F. can be so funny. And I dug out a few old poems to work on as a higher form of verbal activity than crossword puzzles.

I'd better copy my poem on the birds before I lose it.

NOW I GROW OLD

Words leave
Like orioles in August.
You saw him yesterday—that bird is a starling.
The best left long ago
Like the pheasant cocks in their splendor,

As they marched up the border in their Chinese rings,
Treading leaves, hens following.
Remember the day they came in snow
And a rabbit, under the pine, bunched in his fur
Never stirred as they headed
Where they were going.
(Only I never had words plumed like a cock; at best, nearer
his mates.)
Still, better the certainty of sparrows
And the chance of a jay with his great squawk of living—*This
is me*—
Than a fall sky dark all over with grackles flying,
All leaving.
I'm not talking about dying.

August 12

A day I couldn't rise above. I remember the old saw of my childhood about a black dog sitting on your back. I was annoyed as I rarely am by my nurse and then Mrs. R. said, "The hell of a nurse you are. Bump, bump. Bang, bang." I felt an echo inside me. A day of dropping things on the floor, out of reach. I decided none of the poems I was working on yesterday is worth it. What I need is a Jane Austen I've never read. (Not a continuation of *Sanditon*.)

August 13

Today, on the other hand, after a visit from Dr. Brewster, but not because of it, I feel I may finish a few poems and that there are worse, though they may not be good for my digestion.

Hearing "Tea for Two" sung fancily in a way I disliked, was suddenly moved to tears for George, thinking of his expression and his gestures over the sugar cake and how funny it seemed to us to think of his taking one of Susan's cakes to the Land Registry "for all the boys to see" (think of Mr. Clarke Williams and Eric Whellon and all of them).

Later—heard of the death of Edward. I still think it is better to live to 68, playing tennis than to go on and on in a life of invalidism (though that may not have been his alternative) but of course overwhelming for Doris. I am sad for Elizabeth—she hasn't anyone now with the past in common, the far past that is, no one like Susan and Tommy. I think all over again of George's death. "Thank God for a good supper. God bless me. God bless you," I hear the big man saying to his roommate. "Yeah," says Mr. D. Mr. D. reminds me of the laconic Mr. G. who used to live opposite us, with Mr. H. Once I heard a night nurse say to him, "Are you comfortable now, Mr. G.?" Mr. G., "Yes." Nurse, "Aren't you going to give us a smile?" Mr. G., "No."

August 14

Picnic, the house kind. Good dinner, by these standards, and an absolutely perfect summer day, but with a breeze. I enjoyed it, in spite of not getting next to Miss K., who looked sad and lost and really is losing the little sight she had when I first met her. This, followed by a nice entertaining visit from Connie, made it an extroverted day.

I'd like to finish the Theseus poem, hoping it isn't cute or coy. I'm sure it's old-fashioned.

August 15

Strange, how days like this fly, even in a place like this. The morning in exercises and music after breakfast—Serkin today playing the *Pathétique,* washing, hot packs, walking briefly— then lunch, a little working on Theseus (whether to any end or not), a visit to Miss K., cut short by a visit from Bea, and a brief spell out of doors from which I barely got in in time for more hot packs, the parallel bars and now it's time for *Times* editorials and perhaps the *New Yorker* till supper. I am distressed for Mrs. R. who not only can do none of these things but is actively suffering from one of her blind eyes.

Have just read an article on the teaching of history in U.S. that infuriates me. The students are becoming preoccupied with *presentism* of all horrible neologisms and think it "not a practical subject." (This according to a report from the Organization of

American Historians.) Not so practical as changing a tire, no—or I can't even remember the name of the essential thing you put in in electricity—a *fuse*. But as practical as painting a picture, though perhaps not so present. I feel angry enough about it to write a letter to someone, but it would have to be a letter to the world.

Read a story in the *New Yorker* called "The Old-Age Home." It's a journal (Aug. 11) by one Lou Myers and I don't believe most of it. One thing rings true—the conviction that people are stealing things (even Mrs. R. believes that), but even granted that the young man was visiting a mother out of her mind, it doesn't seem there could be quite such a collection of grotesques, left more or less free to dress in the most extraordinary collection of garments. There seems to me also a preponderance of social workers over nurses—nurses are hardly present at all—no one is in charge and far too many deaths in what seems quick succession. In a way there is a kind of genuineness about Ma, but for the rest, it is as if the place were seen through her eyes, not those of the supposedly normal son visiting. There is an unpleasant minor character in it who is "on her head" and reads the Op. Ed. page of the *N.Y.Times*, just like me.

August 16

Heard definitely from her that Sarah is leaving. I regret this deeply. When comes such another? A head nurse here has to take on more responsibility than the head floor nurse of a hospital, who has doctors in every day, and she takes it. One of her young nurses said to me once, "She sets an example to us all," which sounds more conscious and *de haut en bas* than she is. And she is only 26. She brings our medicines later than the people who substitute for her because she stops to listen to everybody's complaints all the way down the hall. She is highly intelligent, express and admirable in action, and, incidentally, beautiful as some Renaissance angel, only we can't quite decide whose. Connie said Fra Angelico, but that isn't quite it.

Another roommate problem: the nurse who was bringing me back from the South Wing was called in by Bill S., who is not clear in his mind (not to be confused with Bill N., who is). He pointed to his roommate of some weeks' standing and said, "*He* got in here."

The nurse kept trying to tell him they shared a room, but he wasn't having any. We left him puzzled, but not belligerent.

August 18

A nice day at home yesterday. Elizabeth talked quite cheerfully of Edward and the church ceremony, and the things said about him—that he managed to be on good terms with everyone in the highly competitive atmosphere of John Hancock, that he cared about how things were said, never rewriting people's letters for them, but getting rid of superfluous words. Good things to have said about one.

Looking at a card of the burial stele of the young woman with the jewels I once tried to write about and am now trying again, I am struck by the superiority of this view of death to the medieval *danse macabre*. She is not being snatched away—nor was the athlete hanging up his garland. Her resignation in the midst of life— beginning to undress after a party?—is complete and beautiful. It is a little different from the child with the doves in the Metropolitan—she hasn't said goodbye to them. She wants to take them with her. (Or is she dressing? I can't quite make out if the necklace is there, round her neck. The box seems closed. I must read more about them. It is just possible the athlete is going to put on his wreath, but I thought not at the time. Elizabeth thinks she is still choosing.)

August 19

Time spent in the hairdresser's chair pleasanter, partly because it was shorter, partly because my mind was still at work on the girl with the jewels and the poem about Delos. I now think I can finish both, by which I do not mean I think them good. I think them not bad and that means my mind runs ahead by habit to the idea of publication. The good thing is that I want to work on them. So I tell myself, wondering if it's any good trying the *Virginia Quarterly* after all these years. Vaulting ambition.

COME AWAY, DEATH

(Greek Burial Steles in the Metropolitan Museum)

Sorrow sits still here: no word or tear,
Where the sad friends come to her chair;
Faces are clear in the gravity of this farewell.
Nothing more still—
The quiet reaches here.

No chill of the dark or the deathbed;
Touch her, she is warm; her bent head
Leans to her necklace or bracelet, to the doves
That alive she loved.
Can they belong to the dead?

Hers is the composure of what is over
Beyond shadow of change. No older
For all her long sitting still, she faces away
From the rising day
And his great, heaving shoulder.

One of my favorite Beethoven cello sonatas this morning (3)
magnificently played by J. du Pré. But our old Janos Starker record is still fine.

August 20

I forgot yesterday to record that Mrs. R. was visited by a gen-
uine admirer out of the old days, a man now 75 and very tanned
and healthy looking. She got a momentary lift, I am sure, and was
pleased when he kissed her. She said her children had put this
man's picture in her luggage when she set off on her second honey-
moon.

Today is a lovely day, with the sun in and out and a feeling of
fall. (But Mr. O. must not say, "Winter's coming.") Elizabeth
came out, the greatest possible surprise and pleasure and we sat in
the sun/shade and talked—partly about India (Dina is over) and
Indira Gandhi and the degree of censorship of the *Times of India*.
Struggled between times with one line of the poem on Boreas at
Delos.

August 21

A black day in our calendar as Sarah has left.

I had a pleasant personal surprise, however, in a visit from Virginia and Nadine, who brought me a different kind of gossip and made me feel for the moment almost gay. They also came bearing gifts, cookies, books, and once again I felt as I did last summer, overwhelmed. Virginia asked what we did about cocktails.

Mr. D. has been moved from his big roommate and put back in the quieter company of Bill N. I hear him protesting to Mr. W.'s daughter that he had never complained. She said, "It was your daughter complained. She said my father was always at you because you didn't pray enough." Mr. D. kept saying, "Say no more about it." She said, "You know my father has to settle everyone's business, but he's 94." She added, "But I still love you." Later we learned she was the one who had Mr. D. moved in with her father. I am amused to think of the embattled daughters. Mr. W. has five of them and one son and the son keeps out of the way—I can imagine past battles. (Or maybe the son has a job in California.) Mr. W. is terribly patriarchal, Mr. D. not at all. Mr. W. seems to reach back into novels about peasants. I am reminded of the Polish woman who was in the next room very briefly (she died ten days after she came in) who suggested grandmothers sitting by stoves, perhaps in Chekhov. Once when they'd got her with great difficulty to the toilet (I was sitting near the door) I heard her sink down: "In the name of the Father and the Son and the Holy Ghost."

August 22

I was thinking—how I got there I don't know, unless by Mr. W., who is like an ancestor walking about—of the ancestors I never saw and how they are frozen, where I know anything about them at all, in attitudes comparable to pictures, except that only James Horner sat for his portrait. I have no image at all of William and ———? Pictersgill, my grandmother's parents. Why did I never ask her her mother's name? That was perhaps because she preferred to talk about *her* grandmother, Grace Joyce Lake, riding to church on a white horse—but where? Oulton? Of my great-grandmother Mary Crossland I have the one picture of her setting out on her elopement on the stage coach, in a red cloak. (Also there is her deathbed, or was it his? His, I think. The scene I put in my novel. That's not a picture, exactly.) My great-grandmother Ackroyd (Mary Barker/Josiah Elmer) whom mother knew and talked of is not a picture to me—except for the brief glimpse of her in her widowhood getting her water, of all places, out of the River Aire. My great-grandmother Clough I knew well in her lively nineties, but her husband (William?) is a blank to me, while *his* father eternally rides over packhorse bridges. So much for my family portraits in a room where I can't even put a thumbtack in the wall.

August 23

Among the bits of and on Donne in my address book, I was pleased to find, "I thank him that brings me a candle . . . that assists me with a spectacle when my sight grows old." I also see, as I look at all the possible starting points in these few scattered notes, of all the books full of others and realize why I could never get started. That, after all, for Donne, is a trifling, incidental phrase, but human, neither thunder nor lightning.

WITH A BOOK OF DONNE'S SERMONS

Our ancestors invited Death
To every feast in bone and socket,
And, seeing life was but a breath,
Carried his picture in their pocket.

Knowing the fact but not the term,
They lay down daily in the grave;
Large on the walls they drew the worm
Amid the shadows of the cave.

How he repaid their interest
We cannot know, or by what mark
He knew his lovers from the rest,
Or how he served them in the dark.

Mr. W., left alone in his room, is singing, whether hymns or Lithuanian songs, I can't tell for the radio, but his voice has carrying power. Much as I'd hate to be in a small room with him, I do pity his loneliness.

Mrs. R. thinks they put eggs in her teapot tonight, as a little while ago she thought they were putting shrimp in her corn flakes. When the news came over the radio of someone (I can't be sure it was a doctor) injecting a paralyzing drug into several patients, she said, "Just what they do to us here."

August 25

Yesterday was my worst day at home, because I could rise to nothing and the excessive wet green closed in on us like life. I felt sodden like the grass, darkened already by the thought of Elizabeth's vacation in September, which I want her to take and which it is essential she should take, and by the question, "How much longer will my knees be able to make it into a car?"

Mr. W. has a new roommate, whom I've not yet seen. I'd like to be able to write a poem on him (Mr. W.), a man like a tree walking, erect, some limbs dead but of great height and girth. Not King Lear of the Steppes—his daughters play rummy with him—but a remnant of a country now gone. Swallowed up in USSR? (I suppose so)—with a fierce life-force, that casts its light or heat like a shadow. I wonder if there are people to whom it gives life? Any of his daughters? I see him at the head of a table, asking a blessing or maybe banging his fist or laying down the law in a tavern, or reading a large Bible in the chimney corner.

August 26

A dull day every way, on which I paid my installments of estimated income tax, and while half-resenting it as a chore, was thankful to have my own power of attorney. I have to ask too much of people now, but it would be worse to have to ask someone—Clarke Lyon?—every time I wanted a new toothbrush. Or worse, to ask this institution, when I have to go on Medicaid (if there is any).

Curious how after my spurt of working on poems, I can't

string two words together or feel it would be worth it if I could. Miss K. told me yesterday that she says Hamlet's soliloquies to get herself to sleep. I found I had two little gaps even in "To be or not to be" and got nowhere with the rest. I'm better on the sonnets and Keats' odes.

August 27

Some of these mornings, after I've gone through the elaborate process of getting up and dressed, I ask what for, what am I ready for?

August 28

If I could paint Mrs. R. and she is still paintable, though less so than when I first saw her, and was struck by the wavy grey hair and its red ribbon, the red robe, the fine bones, and dark eyes— she looks more worn now—I would paint her, with the enigmatic pensive look she has now, though she may be thinking only of the "beautiful home" she has worked all her life for and lost. It looks more complicated than that. She *is* complicated, often surprising one with wit. Anger, even revenge—revenge that can never be carried out—is necessary to her. Yesterday she was down on her stepdaughter after she'd gone and said the things she'd brought—pastry and buns fresh from the baker—were out of her (Mrs.R.'s) old tin—"She didn't bring us anything." It was no good saying either that they were fresh or that I'd seen her taking them out of a bag.

This afternoon outside, listened to two women talking, a patient and a visitor, and shrank from the language (Nixon–White House kind) which seemed to destroy part of the effect of the sun and woods.

Bertile sent me the *Harvard Advocate* that is dedicated to Auden and I find I can't read some of the things said without crying.

He got what he wanted. A coronary, he'd said:
it's quick and cheap.
For him then we should rejoice.

That's Monroe Spears, "Remembering Auden," a long rambling

81

reminiscence. "Forgive this unmemorable speech" is moving, all the same.

Disgusted with my poem on *A Midsummer Night's Dream*, for which I think I have a beginning and end but not the middle. I know what I want the middle to be but haven't the words—I want glimpses of Stratford but not a catalogue and I want the effect of the nights when the moon clears suddenly from a cloud and one sees details—the *what* of foxgloves? I don't want it to be a list of possibilities. The scudding and sailing. But as Auden told somebody (I'm enjoying the *Harvard Advocate*), it's no good knowing what you want to say.

August 29

Simple, difficult conversation with Mr. D. above the radio, but difficult in any case. With Mrs. R.'s help I finally got through to him that I admired his pajamas and he said his daughter chose them. "Nice," he said, "Pink, yellow, grey." Mrs. R. said, "Tell her your neighbors admire them." He said, "The neighbors are nice around here. All but when I got in with that old man. He was like a snake." And I'm sure poor Mr. D. felt like a rabbit in the embraces of a boa constrictor.

Picnic, perhaps our last, as Elizabeth goes off for most of September. Hot sun. No birds. Sarah arrived unexpectedly and we had a nice talk about her job, her husband's, the other Depression we began to teach in, Elizabeth and I, and I was visited with one of the rare feelings of the blessings of age, that one doesn't have to go and look for a job and write the endless letters. I remember especially those I wrote in Canada, supervising prep. and being interrupted every five minutes, to colleges unknown (preferably, I thought, looking out at the snow, below the Mason-Dixon line). Out of all that Hood College emerged, just below the Mason-Dixon and it served.

August 31

It can't be possible that August too is gone. Last August I think I'd just got the sling off my arm, but was full of hope.

What a strange spectacle it must have been yesterday to see

Miss K. and me at the ends of her telephone hearing aid (a great device for conversation) reciting in concert "To be or not to be." We got most of it but I still forget about "the spurns that patient merit of the unworthy takes." She remembered it better than I did. We then recited "Thou wast not born for death, immortal bird." I don't know what her roommate thinks. She behaves as if we were not there. The gods—the kind in "The Lotus-Eaters"—would laugh. Is it a way of convincing ourselves we are still the same person? Anyhow I found it exhilarating, though rejecting the bare bodkin as beyond my powers, and postponing it even if I could use it—and, of course, if I had one. And rejoicing over "the insolence of office."

Reading further in the *Harvard Advocate*, I realized, what I had not known, that Auden's death was the perfect one—he died in his sleep after a poetry reading that was a success. What more could one ask? Jo once said that Professor Saunders had a perfect death, sitting in his chair reading the *N.Y.Times;* my uncle Ernest, known in the family as a "scamp" (and that's a word I have not heard for decades), had another kind—he was out in the early morning, picking mushrooms.

September 3

A day and a night at home. Labor Day was beautiful and we sat out to drink sherry with Jo and admire (at least Elizabeth and I admired) the Northern Spies reddening at the top of Ruth Lawson's apple tree. We had given up thinking that tree would ever produce apples at all, and the fact that we can't reach them and that they are probably wormy in any case doesn't interfere with the sense of triumph.

Two good things today, the weather—blowy and autumnal but warm enough—and Jimmy's return, after pneumonia. Jimmy gives one the same sense of safety as Anna Jane—perhaps Joan, too, will be such a person.

September 4

One of the low days, where one is afflicted with not accidie, perhaps, but a feeling of thick dullness one can't break out of—

anhedonia? Yesterday I took a certain pleasure in paying bills and sending in checks, even, and much pleasure in the air. Today I can't get through to anything. I feel there are layers between me and poetry. I can't even write a letter.

Mr. W., as we sat outside together—that is, no one else was there—"Do you know that fellow down there?" (Mr. H., who was walking down below). I said I did, that I lived opposite him. Mr. W., "He's no good. He's lousy." I said nothing. Mr. W., "Bad with women."

Heard that Mr. T., the dandy of the East Wing (his wife also dresses), has left because of the food. This in Mr. O.'s mouth has become, "He was starving to death." (A member of the staff tells me this was not the reason.) I regret them, as a pair. They belonged to the world—not exactly my world, gayer, but something nearer to it. I began wondering, when my insurance runs out, shall I consider moving to a place where the food is better? But I want to be sure the professional staff is as good. And the food really better.

September 8

Yesterday at home was good. Sitting out seemed almost blessed and serene. The day itself was perfect, there was a crop of rose buds which conceivably may come out and the apples were redder, not Paradisal exactly but truly and recognizably apples and for the moment ours, with no serpent wound round the tree. Whoever has the house after us—and we spent a lot of time talking about our wills—is free to chop it down I suppose. Anyhow we don't have to worry about leaving it to anyone.

Today a return to the realization of our common decrepitude. Someone moaned a lot in the night. Mrs. R.'s eye infection was very bad and she is worn out, transparent and old, asleep as I write after a visit to the eye doctor and no food. Miss K. was feeling cut off because she said her better ear had failed her suddenly and there was no one to turn to. When her sister came in with what she called sad news of the death of a man who was tied to his bed in a nursing home, Miss K. said, "But isn't it good? Isn't he lucky?" It seems no one should ever feel sorry for the death of any person in a nursing home. To have died yesterday in contemplation of the apple tree were to have been most happy. Except of course that we've got to get our wills in order, especially mine.

(Having consigned myself to the grave, and not frivolously, I found myself quite interested in an illustrated article in color on Limoges enamels.)

A nurse told me this morning that it was a toss-up whether I or Mrs. J. was the best-dressed woman in the East Wing. Never having been anywhere near such a height in any place I've lived or worked, I felt a slight lift. Of course, as Elizabeth points out, most people here can scarcely be said to dress at all. I see no one emerging to take the place of Mr. T. as best-dressed man. Denise says there is a man in one of the other wings who dresses—it must be South. (West is all hope abandoned.)

Curious effect of moving from the provisions of a will (we have the appointment with the lawyer) to a poem about Brighton and sitting in a shelter with Mother. I have them both on the table and both on the go at one time.

September 9

Lovely day of warm sun and air fresh enough for coats as we picnicked out on the grass.

Finishing up the Auden volume I came on Anthony Hecht's piece, the only one with any mention of Ischia, and found Auden long ago described himself as "an unmade bed." What I had given Jimmy credit for, someone told me had come from some TV comedian. Perhaps it goes back before that, to the time beds began to be made, whenever that was. I think of the beds at Scarrabrae—certainly nobody ever thought of making those. A. Hecht also said that Auden in those years had a parlor game in which people had to say what they'd do with the last month of life, if they were guaranteed eternal salvation—what novels they'd read, etc. Nothing was said about where they'd spend it, which seems to me most important. I suppose, all being young, they'd never think of making conditions about wind, limb, and eyesight. He seems to have limited it to enjoying one's tastes in the arts for pure pleasure, no self-improvement allowed. He chose the novels of Ronald Firbank, the poems of Tennyson, the overtures of Rossini and the paintings of Caravaggio, which are all very far from being my choices, without my being able to pin my own down. If I had a month I'd want to be able to play Mozart, Bach, and some Beethoven, some Schubert, Handel, Haydn, Purcell, along with a few madrigals. With poetry it's harder. The assumption would seem to be that eternal salvation includes none of these joys. No art, no nature—and yet an awareness of suffering? I wonder what Auden thought would be involved in eternal salvation? Truth without the screens and mists of imagery? Love without persons?

It is distressing to me now to hear Mrs. R. express so much favoritism for one child and such bitterness against the others. She said of Irene, "I wish she were out of my life." I dare say I sometimes wished my parents were, though I never said it. Now I try to write a poem of sentiment about my mother. But I wish Mrs. R. did not have to suffer so from her deep rankling bitterness, so much of it based on misconceptions and so much about things. She can't help loving Willy best—that is one thing. And she may be right about the son who doesn't come to see her. But all the conspiracy etc. only destroys her and it is painful to look on at it. Except that one knows she is cut off from new sources of absorption in life.

September 12

Yesterday at home to make my last will, I feel as if it's a paper will—of course it is paper. Perhaps I should say it's not worth the paper it's written on. All these beautiful bequests will inevitably be swallowed up by some nursing home or other. Nevertheless I feel better to have it made and the young man from Davenport, Millane & Connon was very clear, and very nice. The rest was beautiful, not only sitting out where the apples showed a little redder, a few more roses were in bloom, and a Monarch butterfly paused on a rose for us to admire it, but eating the apple sauce from our own Northern Spies and the jelly from our own grapes. (We'd given them up for ever.) I felt full of sentiment and benignity.

Turning the leaves of a book Mrs. Maxwell lent me (a compilation of aphorisms about living and dying, the idea of which I tend to reject, because you don't get enough of any one thing and also because one suspects a design of uplift), I was pleased to come across Montaigne and his cabbages. That is a death like Ernest Marshall's picking mushrooms. Only I'm sure M. didn't die that way, though I forget how he died. I hope not painfully, of the stone. Rather naturally, I began on the section headed Retirement. None of the people quoted was thinking of a nursing home or of the people kept alive when there is no hope. I suspect the total effect of being too optimistic and of overlooking the writers who'd upset their apple carts, e.g., Yeats. They have an annoying tendency too to say "after ———"; they even change "Beauty is Truth, etc." to something more explicit and say "after Keats." But there are some interesting things—Santayana, poems of E. Dickinson I'd forgotten or never read, though another annoying thing is that they so rarely give a whole poem or even a substantial passage. (William Sentman Taylor and Phoebe L. S. Taylor.)

September 14

Having finished my poem for my mother, or about her*— and had it approved by Elizabeth—I found myself strangled with an emotion or complex of emotions beyond analysis. Nostalgia and guilt only part of it. It was partly the feeling for the way life crystallizes itself, though it may not become art—the poignancy of what is vividly remembered. It isn't a "tears, idle tears" sensation so much as an acute realization of transiency, I think, which wrings the heart, without making one wish to deny or lament it. And I didn't feel these tears were idle. I'd rather have written "The Ode to Autumn" than "Tears, Idle Tears," much as I love certain lines in the latter.

September 15

The return of Dick to the East Wing, amidst universal rejoicing. And no one could be more unself-conscious about his popularity. I am sure he had a triumphal entry as he came down the hall from one room to another.

* See September 20, 1975, entry—Ed. note.

September 16

Bill N. has left, not to go home as he wanted, but for another nursing home. He had to put clothes on nevertheless. I regret his warm smile, which was all I knew of him. Heard the following conversation between Mr. H. and Mr. O. this morning. Mr. H., "The fellow next door—he goes in the toilet and doesn't pull the chain." (Pulling the chain takes one back.) Mr. O., "But he's a nice fellow. And he's going." Mr. H., "He ought to go. He's rotten. He doesn't pull the chain." Mr. O., "He's a good fellow. I like him." And O., who is genuinely social, will miss him, chain or not.

Very nice card from a former student, now a member of our department, in which she said Prose Style had contributed to her idea of good teaching and thanked me for introducing her to a passage of Sidney's *Arcadia*. As she was one of the brightest people I ever had in class and I had her in my last year, I can't help being pleased. I had thought my last year something of a failure.

September 18

Still the same dull, chilly weather with a picnic planned and canceled. Went on a trip to the Cooley Dickinson for a chest X-ray, which will probably show nothing—ordered by the new broom, LePage, who is taking over during Dr. Brewster's vacation. Saw part of the new building, which created all those hideous sounds and tremors with drills under the windows when I was *in* the C-D. It's like going into any new hotel—soft-carpeted, supermarket doors and Muzak in the wall. . . . Joan Fontaine back on the radio, caressing the Arnold two-pound loaf.

> Back to my Theseus poem. *A bit of church I found—*
> *Nothing but   stuff made this moon*
> *Tho   confounded*
> *Which transcends the calendar. It shines now as for all*
> *Tell your hounds (Made of real and solid stuff. Take the*
>   *moon*
> *Outshone the calendar   (Set dogs baying)*

Moon with his lantern
Shadows solid as haycocks   *(Meadows of sweet hay*
    over the rooftops—the B
Tilted the stones of   *the innyards where the moon was*
    drunk
Long ago mid summers of flood lit water one down
Shadows as solid as haycocks, and the
Hedgeflowers brush the face, wet and a fox crown
Maybe a thorny hedgehog.

From all this   *and a multitude of shadows* *

I'm still mulling over the Theseus poem. Writing the above notes I remembered a beginning I'd lost completely about crossing the cemetery in the fall when the ghosts asked what was going on *now*—I don't suppose its loss matters but I'd forgotten it altogether. It ended with starlings, but I could never imitate their imitations.

Going to the hospital for X-ray was driven by Steve O'Connor whose name is called so often over the intercom. A little man who likes to talk about his family, without much variation of face or any drama but he keeps it up—facts mostly. He told me his nephew was to be buried tomorrow, had been swept off a rock into a high sea at Gloucester. Then he said, "My father was drowned in the '36 flood at Hadley. Swept off a boat." I could imagine the horror of the thing at the time—he must have been a small boy. He seemed to expect no comment or reply.

September 20

On this most miserable day, in the dark almost (no one round to draw the curtains even) with all my cold symptoms still intact and unhappy reactions from the antibiotic pills, I will solace myself by copying the Brighton poem into a safer place than it's in now. For what it's worth.

* Draft of unfinished poem. For final version, see July 25, 1976 entry—Ed. note.

SEAFRONT AT BRIGHTON
In memory of I.M.H.

Passing, it was the people passing
Held us together.
Heads in the wind, holiday-making feet striking the concrete
Above the shock and reverberation of the sea-wall.
There was a never a time they would stop
Passing, crossing (though in memory they all go one way)
Families, lovers, dogs,
A mother dragging a child, a child dragging a spade,
Some outlandishly garbed as an offering to Holiday.
Look, we say, in our glass shelter,
There goes—perhaps the bearded man with the poodles,
He lives in such a street, you say, knowing all the dogs.
There's the red woman again—her shoes are killing her.
He's new, the little man with the big wife and the boxer pull-
	ing his arm out.
Silent, we watch a beautiful girl alone,
How she prints the air with her clarity.
But most are interchangeable, forgettable,
Nobody, like us—who nevertheless,
Wrapped in a cloak of invisibility, have our say,
While the sea booms as in a cellar,
Clouds bowl across and the half-crown pleasure-boat comes
	rocking in.
And afterwards, home up the windy street,
Where bows and bays face across area railings.
Afterwards, warming our hands on the teacups,
We make something of the afternoon, add it
To other afternoons yesterday and far back;
We build a shelter, frail and narrow but enough,
While a small flame moves in the grate
And from the street the sound still rises
Of feet passing, passing
And now past

Thinking of the books I ought to be giving away to the young
now, books I *know* I'll never read again. I keep thinking I can't be
sure. Shall I ever look at the *Allegory of Love* again now, when I

haven't these five years? Or C. S. Lewis on the sixteenth century? Or my translations of *The Golden Ass*, Urquart's Rabelais, or that charming restoration comedy translation of *Pluralités des Mondes*? I used to think of retirement as a space surrounded by books and myself as going from flower to flower. The sad thing is that one wants to read detective stories at night, even though only in the last hour before sleep.

Today is one of those days when beds don't get made, wastepaper baskets emptied, when I never got time to brush my teeth and the center light has gone out.

September 22

I am torn between not wanting the summer to go and wanting Elizabeth to come back. Today very disappointing because warm, and yet cloudy with a shower just when I wanted to go out. From all points of view it is so hard getting out these days and it makes me wonder how I can stand the winter.

We have a new inmate called Dotty, which seems an unhappy name for one who is mental in a fey kind of way, with a high voice and laugh and a way of uttering high birdlike sounds. Last night we think she must have untied herself and when she was being tied up again, took to shouting, "Help, help, police." She kept it up a long time. Since we've lost Martha Danielson with her ring of names, to the West Wing, we haven't had anyone who raised so much noise. There is Mrs. P. who calls, "Nurse," or "Jimmy," or "Rich-ard," persistently, but she knows, I believe, what she's doing. She just wants attention. Well, I want more than I get since Sarah left.

There is a man here (young for here, though he has a grandchild; his daughters look young—girls, and all much alike, including the grandchild) who is dying slowly. His family comes in numbers and there are always some sitting outside his door. I think it is cancer of the throat he has and he is kept under drugs most of the time. One niece, a nun not in the uniform of the order, comes often.* I wonder if she prays for his death. I get the impression of a large, religious, and very devoted family. In an old picture they'd

* Wrong. The nun was a daughter, had a uniform. The other a daughter.

be on their knees round his bed. Here they obey rules and sit in the drab, antiseptic corridors while one goes in. I never have spoken to any of them, but two of his sisters who are well-dressed matrons, sociable, hair well-cared for, etc.—they come every day too. But it is the slim dark girls who wring the heart.

In the *New York Review* which had very little in it for me this time, I found a poem by Mark Strand which moved me—"Exiles." And I really disliked him when he was in the department. The dislike rising to a height on the day of the Glascock Poetry Prize cocktail party at our house, when he said, "Can you get a drink in this house?"

September 23

Elizabeth's card about the wildflowers by the beach, somewhere in Maine or New Brunswick, moved me to tears not so much of nostalgia as of *desire.* That is one of my ideal landscapes and no one should live too close to it—one should come upon the beach, with its rocks and wild roses and any sea birds and driftwood. No Daniel Hoffmans to try and tell you it's private.

Cheered up in very low spirits by reading that the Willits-Hallowell Center at Mt. H. promises one "unabated happiness." I thought that was solely within the jurisdiction of heaven.

September 24

A nurse this morning complained that she kept on getting the same patients, one who was always taking her clothes off, one who screamed, "Police!"—and one who fought and bit and scratched. It is hard on these young women. But terrible to think of being reduced to biting and scratching and screaming. And not to be able to say, "There but for the grace of God," as it may happen to oneself, with or without the grace of God.

I suppose the man who is dying so slowly, and I am sure painfully in the hours he can't have the drug, is an example of what one would choose in preference to the hospital method of keeping the body alive. (There's a suit on this in Penna.—or N.J.—at the moment, the parents begging or indeed suing the hospital to let their daughter die, when she is in a coma, and there is no hope of recovery.) I'd still take this way, but it is unbearable for them all that his body clings to life.

September 25

Woke to rain, with the promise of more. There goes my picnic with the Potters. Today Paul has his operation and Connie will be with him. Half the reading group in hospitals, one way or another, the other half on the road in Canada. But we got the G Minor Quintet on *Morning Pro Musica*—I think that would have to be one of my six desert island records, a game they used to play on the BBC. I always marvel that anything can have so much of the sense of tragedy of life in it and rise above it in the last movement. The music was all good this morning—I find I've enjoyed the Chopin series and especially the Preludes.

September 26

The man (Mr. Moriarty) died a few minutes ago. It was strange to realize it by the fact that all of the watchers went away —I'd watched them come in at different times for so long and just now happened to look and see them all going away together, two sisters, two young girls, and an older woman, probably his wife. Someone has been here day and night for what seems a long time —it's been their life and they'll miss it at first. Without knowing them at all, except for an exchange of greetings with the sisters, I have found the whole thing moving, unlike all the other deaths while I've been here. There was something very sad in the little group going away in silence, while up and down the corridor different radios and TVs uttered different sounds, a total din.

September 27

Today a very low point—weather, feelings inside, asthma, minor minimal disappointments, like failing to get my letter to Elizabeth in Nova Scotia and the fact that Bertile did not think my Brighton poem worth commenting on—perhaps it is for the family circle. Having begun to be interested in writing again, I should school myself to the idea, probably the reality, that what I write does not belong to the times.

Listened to a long conversation between Jimmy and Mrs. Hill on the chaos in the kitchen and over the serving of trays that is a result of the new management. And I'd been so much aware of the chaos in the nursing service as compared with, say, the summer. And of course all this coincides with the weather that is not summer, floods of rain, rivers rising, the apple crop spoiling. Summer's over.

Flood warnings out until 2 A.M. Several streets closed.

September 28

At last the rain has stopped and the leaves that have turned yellow behind my back are drifting down in sunlight.

I keep coming back to the man who died, or rather to the mourners. The scene is old, the surroundings new. The privacy of death has been taken away. There were no radios to say I love you and all the other things they are saying one against another, no TVs with the distance of their news from personal loss and their obscene advertising, as they sat there in this long, unlovely corridor —none of this in the old death at home, where I am sure his pain could have been unendurable. I read in the paper that he had two sons—they may have come but I never saw them. It was all women—wife, sisters, daughters. Again the very old scene of "women must weep," though in pant suits. I'd say I'd never forget them going away, turning their backs on the place that had been an everyday occupation—but that I *shall* forget, that and much more.

September 30

Yesterday my nadir so far, chiefly, as I believe, thanks to Dr. LePage's asthma medicine. Today I had a brief sit out of doors, joined by Bea and Jo, followed by a brief visit from Miss K. and managed to pull myself up on the bars, though not brilliantly. I tried to put something down about the mourners, but fear it may be too facile.

94

We never saw him, the man who lay dying
In the bare room like the rest of the rooms, rarely
The one, whichever it was, stayed by his bed, only
The watchers outside in the corridor,
All women, wife, sisters, daughters.

I have seen their like often in Italian painting,
Presences at the edge of some holy death, kneeling
Hooded or coifed in the shadows while the sky opened.
But these wore the garments of Middle America
And sat on narrow chairs in a hallway

With an incessant traffic of vacuum cleaners,
Carts with linens, brooms, pills and elixirs,
While from doorways issued conflicting music
Or smooth confident voices; a thoroughfare
Too open and too unquiet for any sorrow.

We hoped that he in his painful wakings
Could warm himself at the flame they tended
All day, then all night too, unremitting,
A way of life. At the distance of the onlooker
It glowed like a brazier in a cloister.

We knew he was dead when we saw them leaving
Not singly or in pairs as they came, but in a huddle,
One already with the mourning women of the ages,
Hurrying to put behind them the bleakness of the corridor.
I could have wished them a few playing angels.

October 2

After all yesterday got home and sat in the garden with the
apples and a few buds of Crimson Glory. The hawthorne berries
have reddened and the pyracantha looks healthy after two years
of scale. Few birds—one robin, one chickadee. Much good talk.
Much pleasure from the familiarity of things, even though I still
felt the effects of Dr. LePage's evil ministrations. (Today to my
surprise Dr. Brewster turned up and switched everything with a

sweeping hand.) Elizabeth and I discussed the Hammond diary (1846–48) and the engaging young man who wrote it—I felt as I did in reading Emerson's Harvard Journal that the young men, having much more free time than the girls, who after all were for the first time doing things girls had *not* done at all, educated each other, as Newman says they do. Willie Hammond certainly developed a fine, independent critical power. I don't think he admired Hitchcock very much—he was no anti-venenian.

October 3

Hair appointment easy this time. Yesterday turned out to be a sad day for mail. Billie Putnam found some lumps she had had removed were cancerous. Both wrote with a quite incredible cheerfulness, which made me ashamed of my lowness. Today a postcard from Billie which says the specialist sees no need for chemotherapy yet, and I was relieved. All this after their cheerful letter from Montreal and the miracle of their walking so far, he with Parkinson's disease, she after her open-heart surgery.

The other letter which plunged me in gloom was really the beginning of the end of my insurance. A report to be turned in by Mrs. Hill, in which, I am sure, she can make no kind of case for me that they won't call "custodial care." I returned to the useless figuring—then forced myself to stop and play with the poem about the death and the watchers, not that I think much of it.

Took communion again, without knowing why, except that Mr. Montgomery makes me feel that the suffering god, the crown of thorns is a very real part of our lives, even though I can't reconcile him with Nature—like the nineteenth century, and young people of my own days at college. One goes on coming up against it. I heard him giving it to two other Catholics out in wheelchairs in the hall (*other* because Mrs. R. always takes it). They both said afterwards, "Well, it's the same food isn't it?"

October 7

Long silence because of asthma and the drugs and vapors used to stop it—I won't say cure it. Reading Thomas's letter, I note that he says (immediately apropos of a tenor on the Isle of

96

Jersey who thinks he's Amen-Hotep II) phantasizing is the real comforter in life. This seems to me true only of youth, though I am not sure even there of *that*. I'd say fantasy plays a very small part in age, that is, as long as one has one's senses. The real comforter is companionship, with fellowship as a slightly lower grade for the scale of relativeness. The other is great poetry and great music (I don't mention great pictures, as they are less necessary to me but to some they offer what poetry offers me, so I should say *art* I suppose) and after all some painting and sculpture has knocked me flat in my time. In youth one relies on companionship, but doesn't know it. As for art, one is learning. But if I lost what wits I have, heaven knows what direction I might go in. It wouldn't be Amen-Hotep II, though. I don't know enough about him. Actually Thomas probably doesn't phantasize much—he's too busy growing things. I suppose nostalgia takes the place of fantasy in age. (Heaven knows I had fantasies enough, including the recurring one of meeting the completely desirable husband—I never set foot on an Atlantic liner without hoping for that.) That and "Oh! would that . . . ." For instance, I read about footpaths in *Country Life* and wish I were setting out with a pack on my back. But this is very different from the fantasy which still has hope in it. I forgot that another comforter of youth, surrounded by fantasy often, is success. Age has given up the idea of it, except I'd still like a crumb or two of it and I dare say Tommy takes immense satisfaction in the success of his garden. Wanting the Red Sox to be a success (Mr. H.) comes in a different category, yet Mr. H. has almost a passion for watching them succeed—a passion over for most people in the nineties and usually long before that.

October 8

Dr. Brock came. Mountain Day—and I might have gone home but felt too asthmatic at time of decision. Therefore I felt delighted when Elizabeth came out and we sat in the pleasant Mountain Day air, watching jays and hearing a few chickadees. A day that recovered itself.

Too much got down by asthma to write anything to anybody. I never felt more as if I'd given in to the place than yesterday —I say this knowing there are lower circles. The disease and the drugs are like the devil and the deep sea. I sat in my chair (wrong for my knees) with the taste of lead in my mouth and my limbs trembling (all from a series of lilac-colored pills), fell over the edge into sleep or woke to look at Mrs. R. and feel I was doing no better than she, despite my eyesight and university degrees and five extra years thrown in.

Today I rouse myself to read a review of two books on Shakespeare in *N.Y. Review* by J. Barber, one by Frances Yates on magic (and politics) but the kind of hermetic stuff I've never much cottoned to—I like country magic and the "cream bowl duly set," etc. But interesting. J.B. says "magic takes imagination literally." Yes, and the simple stories about three wishes, genies in bottles, etc., are a very elementary form of this; often with cautionary tales added—e.g., I'd know better than to wish simply to go home, and in the tales one is never allowed to make conditions. I remember a story I read in childhood called "The Stump that Spoke," in which the child who was given twelve, not three, wishes—one ought to be able to manage things on twelve—was not allowed wishes like "I wish all people might be kind to one another," so wasted the rest wishing that various people might have rice puddings—I used to wonder why anyone would wish for a rice pudding. (It was a Swedish story by someone called Z. Topelius.) I seem to be straying from F. Yates and Joe Barber and the idea that imagination goes far beyond granting wishes—or charming snakes, etc.—and makes a new heaven, new earth. That is of course in the great. Shakespeare is no genie in a bottle, but whoever (and I'm not sure we know about this in Arabian Nights, etc.) made the bottles, in fact, it doesn't work out. No one *wishes* for what he gives there. Incidentally I suppose there was a parable in "The Stump that Spoke" and the child, whose name escapes me, was a good human being. My first wish at this moment wouldn't be for someone else (world peace wouldn't pass); I'd choose for myself a sudden painless death and I'd say tonight or tomorrow, but would prefer to sign my will first—which no genies would allow.

The Red Sox lost today.

Springfield had a magnificent Columbus Day parade in the rain. The rain was thought to account for the smallness of the crowd under umbrellas.

F. Lee Bailey has talked ninety hours with Patty Hearst (think of him clocking all those hours) and says she is confused.

There was an item on the radio on Rose Dugdale which I missed.

October 14

Yesterday (Columbus Day as now kept, called Landing Day somewhere—Wisconsin?—and Discovery Day in some other states) turned out much better than I expected. Lovely music both morning and evening. Gave up the purple pill. Elizabeth came out and we even sat in a sheltered corner outside and watched the antics—displays of aimless energy—of Jean's children, while the leaves fell and the sun went in and out.

There is a man here, Bill S., who is what they kindly called "confused"—a very solemn-faced man who rides up and down all the time in his wheelchair, without a flicker of expression. Once or twice he has come to our door with something like a smile, and asked us for___?___ . We both struggled to understand him. Last night, while Isaac Stern was playing, a nurse told me Bill S. used to be a violinist in a symphony orchestra. (The Potters knew him and say he made violins also.) This seems to me unbearable. This is not Santayana's "end of a party." I was interested in him before, but because I heard him say to the night nurse when she came to ask if he were all right (he was talking to himself), "Are *you* all right?" And last night when she asked him if he was warm enough, he said, "What about you?"

October 16

Yesterday at home, mixed, but moving toward life. At first sitting in the garden—still some apples on the tree—I wanted to lie down under the leaves (I remember a poem I wrote or half wrote about the surrender of Paris, where we went for water lilies and "I wanted to lie down under the leaves, under the lilies"). This time I wanted a kind of babes-in-the-wood death, with the leaves drifting down. I never saw them fall more gently, casually, detaching themselves without a sound, like dying in sleep. While the trees, our trees, still looked full and round, the maple red, the dogwood dark rose, the poplar still yellow, not the papery white of the same kind of poplar in the valley. I thought of "Call for the robin redbreast and the wren," which I took to be a sign I didn't really want to die that minute.

The Putnams' cheerfulness and sensibleness also made me ashamed of my half-aesthetic self-pity. Bill with Parkinson's disease advancing, Billie with cancerous cells, their son whose letters I read, building and planting in spite of almost certainly fatal cancer. But I came into the living room to find Bill asleep and was shocked to see how much he looked like a deposition from the cross—the worn face, the beard.

Bertile reminded me of the words I only half remembered, "O ye seas / floods / dews and frosts / stars of Heaven! and whales, bless ye the Lord." (I couldn't remember anything but the whales. Those were my favorite Sundays in church when we sang that.)

October 17

Pure misery of a head cold on top of asthma, a little lightened by thinking of the leaves coming down in the garden and wishing I could write about it lightly, like Herrick, lightly I mean in the sense of hardly touching it, getting the effect of the silent severance, as if *this* were the time—no waiting for storm or port, no thrashing of branches.

October 19

All these days are misery, with steady rain and cold, and congested nose and ears, and the feeling that I *can't get out*, can't get anywhere where I could get over the perpetual feeling of wretchedness, chill, anhedonia.

Yesterday witnessed another brief, nasty family scene—this time between Mrs. R. and the daughter-in-law she was on excellent terms with when I came. Mrs. R. was completely unreasonable, but I suppose it is wrong to expect it. She said she didn't want the cookies Lydia brought, then when she complained the radio was wrong (it wasn't) and Lydia suggested taking it, Mrs. R. said, "You're not taking my radio—you've had everything else." (Or something approaching that.) There was more—something to do with arrangements for Mrs. R. to get to the oculist, in which she made it clear Willy was the only one who cared for her. At which Lydia said, "I'm sick of this damn family," and departed abruptly. I can't blame her, but Mrs. R. has got herself really to believe they've all robbed her but Willy who is buying the house back. What I'm afraid of is that she'll be left with him alone, with his unreliable health and the certainty that he can't take her and care for her.

October 20

One thing I note since I became more and more preoccupied with my physical feelings is that I write less about the nursing home, more about myself, less too of the state of the world, which indeed is harder for me to reach and less susceptible to letters to one's congressman. I want to put down my babes-in-the-wood poem, which I'd really like to be sung.

WORDS FOR MUSIC

Come without sound
Now, while the leaves float brilliant
Through the air
Down,
As the leaves noiseless part from the tree,
Come to me,
Not with the apple's commotion,
The thud in the grass, or the late shut roses'
Slow inward decay,
Let the last life-thread whatever it be
Give way
With the leaves' lightest severance,
So, on such a day,
Now.

Do not wait for the wind and rain
Thrashing, the boughs' crack and rending,
But on silent final wings, landing
In the garden where we began,
Come
This stillest day of fall—
Leaves in the air, leaves still on the tree
Leaves to cover me.

October 23

Last night the Red Sox lost the World Series. I do not care, but was brushed by the general excitement—one of the nurses who'd backed Cincinnati running round long after her shift was over to collect her bets. Mr. H. took it very quietly. I wonder if he is lost now or if his walks in woods and finding of wormy apples, etc., will make up. I, being in a state of thick congestion, would give much to walk in woods and find the wormiest apples.

A visit—we've had one or two before—from a girl at UMass, visiting us as part of a class in psychology without any notion of what she was supposed to be looking for. This strikes me as typical of UMass* and indeed of many modern courses outside the UMass; you go out to do something *real*, like visiting an old people's home. I put her through it trying to get out of her what she would write up about us. "Oh!" she said, "it's just a general psychology course. It's really the same course we had in high school." When I pushed her, she said, "Oh! I don't think we *write* anything." As she didn't ask what she could do for us, I got her to water my plants. Mrs. R. and I both worked harder than she did, telling her what she might say. She didn't ask us a single question.

October 25

Yesterday another beautiful day at home, the last we'll have sitting out with leaves on the trees—a few and still falling. Jo was with us and quoted "Margaret, are you grieving / Over Golden-grove unleaving." Jo took me round the cemetery too, to see his

* I later found it was Springfield Technical College.

tombstone—we all have our own ways of luxuriating in our deaths—and I admired the beautiful stone-cutting, and then when we passed another one, already occupied, Jo delighted me by saying, "Old Gondolf with his paltry cornerstone." Thank God for the consolations of our profession.

October 26

The worst fight of all so far. Mrs. R.'s will—I will *not*—and impotence against some professional knowledge and a certain amount of patience that gave out. The fight was partly the usual one about putting on clean clothes, partly the sterilizing of her skin before they gave her the heat lamp for a bed sore—"You can't put that on me. I'm allergic to everything." All this with much "Jesus, Mary, and Joseph" and some Nixon language. Curiously, at the end of all this, Mrs. R.'s eyes were bright—with the consciousness of having asserted herself? While I felt like a rag. The nurse was out to assert herself too.

Have just read that Nixon at San Clemente seemed vital and vibrant to visitors.

October 27

Yesterday continued right up to the evening, when Mrs. R. sent for Willy and begged him to take her home. She was frantic—one felt torn in two, as I'm sure her son was. This morning, when a gentle, experienced nurse gave her the lamp treatment, without a murmur from her, I thought of the terrible self-assertiveness of the young that is different from the futility of the "No, No, No" of the old—it was "I'll show you who's master," and that seems to me utterly wrong for a nurse. Also rare in my experience. (Millie here today.)

October 30

If Mass. goes bankrupt—the possibility is aired in tonight's papers—then we may be indeed in the position of those Cambodian refugees one saw carried on the backs of their sons and grandsons. Whose back should I be carried on? I have been more depressed physically and, so, mentally, the last two days than I can express. A weariness and an irritation with the place seemed insupportable because I realized I am on the side of those who will stay, those without hope—Mr. D. cruising about despondently in his wheelchair—and not those who are learning to walk, improving, the hopefuls of the therapists. It suddenly came over me with a wintriness like today's landscape—three or four flakes wavering down, dark clouds, no color—that there was nowhere to go from here. A visit from Dr. Brewster did not encourage me at all.

November 4

Most of the time between this and the last entry—all but going home—a continuation of the same physical depletions and mental lowness, chiefly from my body's behavior but also because of remarks overheard, which made me feel a little as I did in the Anne S. period, except that *that*, hostility, coming from an intelligent person, in such a form, was nearer the bone and almost unbearable at the time. Mary N. in her letter yesterday said, "We are never ready for our infirmities." I thought I had accepted mine, to find I am not ready for the extra ones, nor ready for the fact that people would change toward me, perhaps because I have become a nuisance. I ought not to be here, my friends say. I ought not to be here, say my—shall I call them enemies? Not to be able to get out and yet to have people anxious to be rid of one is a dilemma I do not know how to rebut. Meanwhile Ford dismissed his more intelligent and respectable advisers and New York City moves nearer to the edge.

November 6

Conte disappoints me by coming out for Ford's reelection—"disappoints," in fact, is mild.

For myself, I feel that I could prowl the corridors restlessly like Mr. O.—only of course if I could prowl I'd go home. I feel less far down, perhaps, but more restless, as if I have nothing to settle to. The "colder looks" are especially apparent to me today, but this may be a pathological thin-skinnedness. Yet some, at least, is real. Suddenly everybody is saying, "There ought to be some way you could live at home." There ought, but I don't see one.

We think of the key, each in his prison
Thinking of the key, each confirms a prison

Last night, Mr. H. came in, when we were in bed, and said—of his roommate across the way—"Look at his feet, sticking out. He doesn't know how to cover himself up. Now I'll have to go and cover him up. I cover him up nice." What is the short story that ends "Well, we are all poor devils"?

November 14

First snow, not settling, but cold enough. A student, who gave me a bath, swept my watch off the table and stopped it. She said, when I said it was not going, "It's probably overwound." A bitter day for the spirit. I can't remember what happened to Mr. Despondency's daughter, but that is a good name for me today. Humiliation is worse than pain. That is, any pain I have so far experienced. I am sure there is excruciating pain that is beyond my knowledge as yet—I think of all the people who have had chemotherapy. The worst of an experience like this is that one keeps hoping it will go away and that is no way of dealing with it. Bertile in a very good letter yesterday said, "I am convinced we are in the hands of God." If I were, I am sure I could rally what forces I have, which aren't much. It may be they are right about my bed's being wanted. They are wrong in treating it as a family situation. Maybe I'll read Bunyan again.

November 18

Nothing improves, though for a moment yesterday and at home on Sunday, I thought it had, or I had. I do not think the remedy is in going to things or learning to make mats. (Mrs. Henderson, who is in charge of all that, came to see me yesterday and told me I could make really pretty things, if I let her show me the way.) I also feel a great heaviness at the thought of all these pressures to come—the sight of the same Thanksgiving decoration, at the front door as I passed it yesterday, opened a vista of years of it, years of Santa Claus and the blind accordion player, while the weariness of the flesh increases. To think I was pluming myself a little while ago on my patience and, worse, enjoying the sensation of being rational in a community in which general ideas are few. At the moment I haven't a scrap of Olympianism and, sadly, very little feeling for the people worse off than myself, whose ills when I first came used to lie on my chest when I heard voices crying in the night. If I could get back—but all I can achieve is " 'Let me out,' said the starling."

November 19

Another visit from the psychology student, as bird-witted as ever, and as hard work. She wants to be a physical therapist because "Not everybody is a physical therapist" (true of all professions) and she is writing a paper on hydrotherapy for her freshman English course. That is a subject I never had offered. Then she thinks this volunteer work may help her to get into the physical therapy training, "if they think I get along good with patients." She does get along good with us after her fashion, in that she is amiable and smiling and willing to talk about herself, though not of course about us. She got 93 in one course, which shocks me. She has a kind of prettiness, with a warm smile and dark elf-locks and a habit of waving her hands. I'm sure someone will marry her.

Emerged from my cloud at least long enough to get indignant with the President over New York as I read the editorial in the *New Yorker*—a wayward daughter, indeed!

November 20

Reading *Country Life* found the old walker in me stirred by an account of the Whin Sill, of which I'd never heard—it seems to be mainly in Northumberland, but touches Yorkshire and the Pennine Way follows it for a while. It is 200 million years old—the kind of fact that still floors one. Now I feel I'd rather be able to walk the Pennine Way than go to Vienna, the unvisited city I most regret. (I remember that when Mrs. Hazelip thought she was dying, she kept saying, "Here I'm dying and I haven't seen Venice," and then she recovered and they took her—a really satisfying story.) It may be that the Pennine Way would always have been too much of a scramble for me as I am sure the Appalachian Trail would, but I was never happier than setting off for the day with a rucksack. Well, I'm glad I walked as much as I did before the cars took over and the arthritis got into my legs.

November 28

Impossible to write because of the prison of self, with little thinking of the key. There is no key—only news from a window. Interesting review in *N.Y. Review of Books* of books on G. Eliot and Hardy, especially the part on Hardy. "Hesitation before life, a lingering around death" and he (Michael Wood) compares H's halfway response to life to the twilight Tess liked to walk in, the moment of suspension, neither day nor night "leaving absolute mental liberty" (H). And "At its best Hardy's pessimism is too nervous and energetic to be gloomy. It tests our comfortable commitment to continuing our daily existence from the point of view not of a potential suicide, but of a living ghost, a man who survived to the age of eighty-eight without greatly caring for Life." At the moment I feel a living ghost, without a ghost's invisibility—"living and partly living." But having, I think, greatly cared for life in my time.

1976

January 12, 1976

It is strange I want to begin again today, with the snow falling steadily and the sense of isolation acute. I think fleetingly of last January when I was at the height of my power and pride; I remember showing off to my visitors—how well I could walk, how I could even climb the stairs. At that time I never doubted I'd soon be home to stay. But I'm not dwelling on it. Meribeth described this January as "ordeal by cold"—at least we are out of that. Over the radio come notices of this and that meeting canceled—hundreds of confirmation classes it seems, the ecclesiastical year moving toward Easter. There is more snow to come but at least we are three weeks past the solstice and there will be more light.

I do not know what to say of the months past, what to pick out. The images fade so fast. There have been changes in this neighborhood, a death next door of one of the people I talked to—a quick death from angina. In her place, they have moved in what at first seemed a mad woman from the State Hospital—she kept up an incessant sort of lolling, in which few words were distinguishable for the first twenty-four hours she was here, all in a voice like a man's. I walked out in the corridor to see her and was shocked to see her tearing at her clothes with bound hands, with her hair loose over her shoulders like a stage maniac. Since then they have quieted her and tidied her up. She is over 90. From lingering death, good Lord deliver us. Instead of the snatching bone and socket figure of the frescoes, I see Death hanging about and waiting, leaning against the wall with his hands in his pockets. Not that he ever had any pockets. Meanwhile our opposite neighbors go on. Mr. O. comes every day, gentle and benevolent, to ask us how we are, are we hungry, what will there be for dinner. I value his good will. And Mr. H. goes on feeding his birds in spite of snow, ice, and all the other horrors of this January. He also always comes to wish us good night.

Incidentally, speaking of Death, as I was, I find *Prime Time* offers me the attractions of both *Death and Dying* and *Images of Aging* this month. Of course what *Prime Time* offers me is one thing and what I get is another, considering the behavior of Channel 57 on my TV set. I'll probably get neither. The programs I don't get have come to seem to me like other people's travels. As to those two programs, I don't need to learn to accept the idea of death (I think)* and I know about images of aging. I'd much rather be able to see *Washington Week in Review*.

Have just read that Nixon marked his 63rd birthday by the most pathetic exhibition of presidential relics in a small museum —pens used to sign documents, the desk Brezhnev sat at, book matches with his name, cuff links with the presidential seal. What a hunger and thirst after fame. I can't imagine how anyone would want to go and see it.

January 15

A letter from young Marie Clifford, who is evidently answering the letters written to F. Clifford about Edna's death. She enclosed a picture of Cedar Cottage under snow, very beautiful, but not as I'd ever seen it, of course. I found myself very much moved by the sight of it, the thought of Edna as the warm center, the hours of sunlight and salt air and pure physical happiness I'd had there, from the first summer when I spent all my time (wartime)

---

* Maybe dying. What I want is to be snatched away from the dance—dance not being the word now, however.

with the boys age 6 and 9 sitting down at the cove while they sailed boats, or following—and once making—trails through the woods. I think it was the next year I was a plane-spotter with Percy at Hiram Blake's—I may say we spotted very few. The cottage with the snow on it was a picture of the end of something about which my tears for myself can have no bitterness. For Ferd Clifford it isn't a picture—he has to go on living in that house alone, lucky only in the fact that the boys had no ambition but to live as near to their own doorstep as possible, so that now he has his children, his daughters-in-law, his grandchildren all within a stone's throw. I heard of E.C.'s death a few weeks ago, but somehow it was the picture of the house in the snow that made me mourn for her. I wish I could remember—that is, put into words—the soft voice, never raised, however exasperating the boys might be, the unhurried way she could throw another piece of wood on the stove, mix a cake, talk, and answer the telephone, while one visitor after another came in, to sit on their hard kitchen chairs and get all the news of the Cape. She kept on being elected Ceres at the Grange, but she was always Ceres, as Elizabeth said the first time she went there with me—giving and giving. And at the same time knowing every boat that came into the dock, every car that went up the road. But I can't write about her.

Our Lady of the Angels has just postponed its evening of Bingo because of the snow.

January 18

This house under snow-light was once my pastoral of summer.

But I think I wrote about the essence of summer feeling in the *mille-fleurs* meadows poem, though I never managed to get down anywhere the feeling of strenuousness and wildness that stout Cortez discovers—though reduced to a hundredth part of the real thing—e.g., of the first sight of Ames's Cove, reached only by slithering down under tough resistant branches, the joy of having it to oneself. The sand dollars. Or the first sight of the cellar hole when we approached Redman's Beach through the woods, and found the remains of the old farm—apple trees and orange lilies. It was all so different from my walks across downland grass in England. When one was alone—and more often I was not—it was much more numinous.* (And here am I without either a memory or a dictionary.) But it's Edna I'd like to write about.

January 20

Snow. A picture of a crow in the *Audubon* magazine fascinates me—large, close, black and blue back with a white eyelid or eye-ring, still—bent-in claws. I see what Ted Hughes saw in it, but how he got close enough I don't know. It may well be the last species left to pick up the bones of the race. There was also a description of its antics in the wind which reminded me of Gilbert White on jackdaws—sheer fun.

The feeling of the toylike outlines of Cedar Cottage as if a child had drawn it, the simple construction of adding a room and a staircase and the woods at the back door, the sounds in the night —an owl killing something perhaps—in the midst of the extraordinary quiet. In those days no one ever locked a door. The cold night we stepped outside and saw the Northern Lights.

Here it isn't only that the nurses talk about bowels, as they have to, the patients talk about their bowels to each other.

Outside it is snowing again. The inner weather is troubled too in this room, though finally the bed has got made. Mrs. R., after a bath, sits and glowers. At times there is just a hint of the Cumaean Sybil in her face, but more suppressed rage. In these isolated days, for all her extra years and blindness, she is a caged tiger. I am a caged rabbit. (Have just read *Watership Down*, where I found I enjoyed the company of those high-toned rabbits, but perhaps even more the downland flowers, thyme, clover, etc., the closeness to the earth. But one had accepted the rabbits'-eye view without which the thyme and clover wouldn't have been enough and one accepted it because he can tell a story.)

January 22

Went not exactly against my will, but caught off guard, to a musical entertainment that was the most interesting I've heard

* It took me a quarter of an hour to think of it.

here yet. The man and wife, in their hillbilly clothes (that may not be the word) had a feeling for their kind of music, which means for music, and had what looked to me to be rather good instruments —guitar, banjo, mandolin, and violin. I cared less for their little girl (pretty enough) who climbed up on a chair and sang and bowed, with too much of the professional. So between that and Mrs. R.'s delight in it and a visit from the always welcome Reverend Mr. Montgomery, I find a lot of the time has gone without my yet feeling sorry for myself on this day of blowing snow when it is 9° at 3 P.M. with a "wind-chill factor of -35°. . . ." There was something moving in the mixture of family feeling with feeling for their job as entertainers, which puts it a bit low. The wife was, perhaps, the entertainer, the man something more of the musician. He sang a song of his own based on a bumper sticker he'd seen out west: "We are all God's children. Call home"—cheap enough, in a way, like that placard Muriel's friend used to carry on his car "You couldn't care less? *He* couldn't care more," except that the "Call home" one seems to me to have more imagination. Anyhow I was touched by the song. As Miss K. says, "A little religion helps around here."

The day ended with the sad news that Dick is leaving to go to a rehabilitation center in N.H., for children. Of course he'll be excellent at the job and will love N.H., but they won't get anyone who'll come near replacing him, as they will learn. I feel inadequate to speak of his "loving and giving" along with a gaiety of spirit that made light all the trouble he was taking, the time we were taking, or the way he brought life and energy into a room with him—"comfort and joy."

January 29

The gentle sad Mr. D. died this morning, after the stroke a few days ago—he never spoke again or ate anything. I have seen him cry twice, once when he was alone in his wheelchair in the corridor, cry openly and it seemed unself-consciously out of hopelessness and loneliness. The other time was when his daughter came—the good daughter who visited him almost every day. He wept when she appeared and said, "You never come." She said, "Pa, I missed just one day, don't you remember?" I am glad he has no more of these long days. Not that I have found them long yet, except for the hour or so of no light in the late afternoons, but he couldn't see well enough to read. He may not, in any case, have been a reader. He had been a barber, but he was not the talkative gossipy type one associates with the trade. A quiet, self-effacing man, wishing, I think, to communicate more than he could with us, his neighbors.

January 30

Thank goodness "Bloody January" is almost gone. A dreary, deflating, dividing month. Some days I have felt an unbearable lethargy, when I wasn't coughing or gasping, that made it seem hardly worthwhile to reach out for the things one might read—all kinds, in a pile on the radiator. There are also things I can't reach which are an intermittent irritation, like dropping things on the floor.

February 1

So far looks just like January, which indeed had its brighter moments toward the end, though it never got much above freezing. Today is wet and grey. Read in an article on concentration camps (Terrence des Pres in *Harper's*) that there was something in the physical act of getting up every morning that renewed hope and life, the will to survive even there in those unspeakable conditions—"from withdrawal to engagement, from passivity to resistance." I find the same thing here in circumstances which cannot be compared with those. There is a kind of triumph in getting up, or having got up every day. Yesterday because I was hauled out early and the sun was shining, put in several hours of *work* for my income tax, almost enjoying the adding up of the vast sums I've spent to stay here. Today because no one hauled me out I lay and listened to Mendelssohn's *Elijah* with some pleasure, but of limited kind. The voices could not have been better, but I found a monotony in the work (cf. Handel) and nothing like the pleasure of interreaction of voices and accompaniment one gets at its height in Bach. Reading *The Golden Notebook* with divided pleasure, and can't follow her when she says novels are dishonest* in foreseeing the end in the beginning and that one ought to be able to put down one day exactly as it happens, which she does, inserting even the menstrual tampons. If I put down all the details of a day here, I'd put myself to sleep writing it.

Last night Mrs. R. told me I was mistaken, she'd had only one husband. I am afraid her sense of time is slipping, as mine may have in five more years. But that is quite new; she had always given me a strong impression of the superiority of her second marriage, as well as a vivid picture of her twelve years of widowhood between the two and the hard work of bringing up her children.

February 3

A long power outage, still not mended. For me the worst thing is not being able to get out of my chair without being pulled out. The worst, that is, so far, though I'll mind if it goes on, with no light tonight—no reading, no radio. Also the meal at noon was cold, not a cold meal but a hot meal inadequately heated. Cold noodles. Visit from Dr. Brewster who annoyed me by worrying far more that I couldn't get Channel 57—he kindly told me all the things I was missing, as if I didn't know—than about my collection of symptoms and complaints. Outside a high wind, which is the cause of the power failure, snow and ice—all winter's miseries over again, when we were hoping for an interlude. The light and power came on after ten hours, so that at least one could read in bed. The radio came on to tell us that in Westfield, where the blackout still prevailed, people could take their bedding and food to certain appointed places, so we felt we had escaped again. I don't know whether the visit of the priest, blessing Mrs. R.'s throat with crossed candles had anything to do with it . . . but our next-door neighbor, an ex-librarian who has been here only a short time and whom I've stopped in to visit occasionally, died last night after a day of gasping for breath which was very audible here. She was very unhappy and I had judged her, I'm afraid, for

* She later retracts this; it was an experiment only.

complaining about her symptoms when I went to see her. It reduces my complaints to the size of pinheads.

I gather that today I have the will to live or I would not put cream on my face. . . . Mrs. R. is convinced her son put an end to the blackout last night. She said, "I called my son and ten minutes later the lights came on." She forgets he was himself in a blackout at E'hampton when she called him. I find such adoration touching and out of my experience. The only thing is it leaves everyone else nowhere.

February 5

I am copying a prayer which Judy, the Yorkshire nurse, got for me—it is in the family prayers of the U.S. Book of Common Prayer: "O Lord, support us all the day long, until the shadows lengthen and the evening comes, and the busy world is hushed, and the fever of life is over and our work is done. Then in Thy mercy grant us a safe lodging, and a holy rest, and peace at the last." (At Night.) I wonder if it was ever in the Church of England version, at the time when they had family prayers, for instance. I note that the 1945 U.S. version from which I copied it had nearly everything the same as my English one, undated but George VI.

February 7

Active morning of bath, then Mr. Montgomery's church service, where I found the playing of the hymns as we sat and waited very moving. "Lead kindly light" is always complicated for me by the memory of Newman's experience in Sicily and the utter strangeness of the bull at Segesta (was it?) and the long fever in a country place where he couldn't speak a word of the language, all somehow working alchemically to project his conversion—then "Lead, kindly light." I should miss hymns in the R. C. service—they go back in me to Lofthouse Chapel, through school and college, becoming rarer in my working life as I went to church less and less, but I feel they're in the bottom layer of me.

I hear our present flu virus is called A-Victoria and there is no serum for it. Several of the nurses have or have had it.

Have begun the *Book of Sansevero*, having read the third volume a year ago and having had to wait for the library to get this. There is something in Giovene's dense, reflective style that is very agreeable to me and I am fascinated by the alien life of the ducal palace and the monastic school. It is odd to read it after, even overlapping with, *The Golden Notebook* with its undiscipline, sex, psychiatry, communism—the 20th century, the post-2-World-War 20th century. (Giovene was born the year I was, into a life bound to vanish.) I enjoyed *The G. Notebook* enough to read it, while feeling a personal antipathy to Doris Lessing along with a respect for her honest, adult observations on life. I enjoy her perception of the ways, by words, people hurt one another. I believe her absolutely on the states of mind of the communist intellectuals of the thirties and their later disillusionment with Russia. Perhaps I enjoyed the conversations with the psychiatrist as well as anything and she is the most sympathetic character as far as I am concerned, though I fear psychiatrists as a race. But I'm interested that Anna's dreams resemble myths. I'm sure mine don't, unless the wandering in the city is connected with the Labyrinth. (I don't have it much any more.) In general there could be nothing much farther from Giovene's shut, austere persona than the uninhibited speech and ways of D.L.'s people, except that both move in the world of ideas. Rather naturally, I like the notebook idea and all the observations on writing in D.L., especially the way a character moves off from oneself. Oddly enough, Giovene also kept notebooks in his adolescence, though with monastic parchment covers and monastic script. His were classified *Aphorisms, Observations,* etc. He could have been a little frightening, with his formidable intelligence and habits of isolation and self-discipline, but that he was surrounded by people who almost didn't notice him.

Mrs. R. and her nice malapropism, "the priest with his acelots." There is something so Bacchic about it. It seems particularly funny with this heavy, thick-lipped somewhat leathery priest, with his perfunctory blessings.

February 10

Finished *The Golden Notebook* last night, as I struggled for breath. The last episodes I found boring, as if we'd had all this be-

119

fore, though I'm sure that was my inexperience and lack of interest in the nuances of sexual relationships. She makes me realize that I value discipline, something she seems to value only in craft and art. Perhaps another reason she's not my cup of tea is that she is so nonliterary—here at least. And as far as I can make out no one ever goes to the theater or to a concert. Marx and Engels, but who else? Even the rabbits had their saga.

Note in passing from Giovene (pp. 136–37) when the narrator goes to sit under the dome of Santa Maria degli Angioli on the way to a difficult interview. "From up there descended blessedness and peace. The impressive shape surrounded all things, brought them back to itself, left nothing outside that was errant or lost." The "errant or lost" part brings in something else, but otherwise I couldn't help thinking of V. Woolf's oblongs and squares and "very little is left outside."

February 14

(Yesterday did *not* get my hair done, the flu having struck down the hairdresser along with so many others. The day before, however, got my toenails cut.)

Price and Pride, the A&P allegory, ceases to be allegory altogether when presented on TV. As a matter of fact *Price* is a difficult idea for allegory in the first place and *Pride* has too many ancestors that belong to the days when Pride was a deadly sin. But to see them reduced to two rather coarse, white-aproned A&P salesmen takes away the generalizing force of allegory. I raise a question here about the deadly sins in Piers Plowman, gluttony in the Tavern, for instance. But he still remains an Absalom in concrete surroundings. Price and Pride are nothing but A&P salesmen, in their habitat. Price I can't fit into any allegorical scheme at all.

Complaint in *Times* on "Cronkitese"—a form of BBC-ism. The writer confuses dialect with accent, however, in complaining that Dan Rather, etc., do not speak their native dialect. Real dialect (Fred Graham hasn't given up his southern accent any more than Sam Irvin).

Notes on popular songs that come over Mrs. R.'s radio. There is more open reference to sex than I had thought—"Lay your head on my pillow / And your warm and tender body close to mine" and "I'll eat your strawberries and drink your sweet wine" (quite Elizabethan). But the references to its being all over are thick, ranging from "the feeling's gone and I just can't get it back" to situations of long standing in which the light has been left on the stairs in case she ever comes back. I notice too an unexpected vein of sentimentality, one of the worst being "Daddy, don't you walk so fast" (a little girl, I *think*, when her father was walking away from it all), but also a cropping up of angels—in one on the loss of a wife (I take it)—"When I was not at home, the angels came"—here a sound of angels singing in the background. In another, the angels conspire to make a dream come true (the girl in question), for all the world like that sentimental ballad of my youth, "Sure, a little bit of heaven fell from out the sky one day," which the angels when they saw it named Ireland, "because it looks so peaceful there." Highly unprophetic.

Today we have hearts everywhere, stuck on whatever can be used to stick things on. A strange demented woman, a new arrival next door, came in here and tried to talk to us in Lithuanian (she seemed to want Mrs. R.'s bed) and I noted that her family had pinned on her a white ribbon, painted or printed with Valentine hearts.

Speaking of Lithuanians, I heard Mr. W., with whom I sat out in the summer air, had died suddenly over in the South Wing. It is too bad they could not have talked together.

February 18

The influenza epidemic, which has been laying out nurses right and left, closed schools and closed most hospitals to visitors, has touched this room, I hope lightly. For me I suspect it is taking the form of a common cold; which seems like another layer between me and the world. Elizabeth today begins on her long session with the Admissions Office so that I shan't be seeing her. Added to which it is snowing again. . . . The Lithuanian, who seems very spry, continues to wander in and out of other people's rooms, lying on their beds if they are not there, like Goldilocks. She is aggressive and argumentative, very voluble, but with no English beyond "I look for my son" or sometimes it is her brother. (Meanwhile Dotty, who has taken the place of Martha Danielson, though with a higher almost a childlike voice and with a much smaller collection of names, calls "Momma, Momma" and, sometimes, "Grandpa.")

February 25

Over the weekend Paul A. died, aged 96, so now there'll be no more of the nightly walks around the building to see that it was all in order, no more "Go home, Paul," "Turn around, Paul," or, sometimes, "Marchez." Lately he had puffed and blown a good deal, walking, and gone through the motions, mechanically it seemed (he walked like a mechanical toy wound up) as if he remembered less clearly what it was he was here for. It is a long time since I saw him with a broom.*

Next door a new woman has moved in with the Lithuanian, highly cantankerous and vocal. I heard her say to a nurse, "I'm 71 and I'm not used to taking orders from a girl like you." She beats with her spoon on the table when she can't get anyone's attention. She is saying already, after less than twenty-four hours, "I'm getting the hell out of here."

To the note on fear of death—in the Middle Ages there was hell of course in the flesh. But the *danse macabre* also shows death coming for the young, the knight and squire, the ploughman at the plough. Death loses all terror—or most of it—in a nursing home. Frescoes don't show him in a lazar house.

February 28

Yesterday I put my face out of doors for the first time since Christmas Day. Anna Jane took me out in bright, warm sunshine along the road by the dam to Chesterfield, a road I've never seen before except with the leaves falling, then fallen, always with some of the color of fall. Yesterday was beautiful even with the

---

* Mr. H. (93) said, "I hear the old man's dead." It is strange that one will miss him and the commotion he created. I am sure the fathers of the French church gave him an honorable burial.

dirty snow patches—ice on the reservoir, but with some dazzling open water, the trees grey—blue—a few maple sap buckets (but A.J. said they looked as if they's been out all winter), almost no one about. I felt especially grateful to A.J. for coming, as she goes every day to the Holyoke Hospital. Aunt Winnie is dying, slowly, still in possession of her mind, and even of her humor. She is a very special person, utterly unaggressive or egotistical. She has true humility and almost nobody has.

March 2

Next door now we have a strange pair, the voluble wandering Lithuanian and the cantankerous woman called Jessie equally voluble who still wants and wants and beats on—it sounds like a tin tray but can't be. (It reminded me of Arcadia and Aunt Grace beating on a tin pan the time we had a swarm of bees.) Last night I heard one of the nurses say to the Lithuanian, "Talk English," and she replied, "I won't." I heard Jessie say, "I'd commit suicide if it weren't for my sister," and a girl who was clearing the trays say to the other one, "But they don't commit suicide." I imagine no one here knows how. Mrs. R.'s threat is always, "I'll go and jump in the river," she who hates a bathtub.

I hear Jessie has already demanded to see the manager, the director of nursing, the head bookkeeper (heaven knows why) and the kitchen manager. Whether any of them came I don't know. She yells "Nurse" at the top of her voice, when she isn't banging on something. She says, "I'm not used to a place like this," as if all the rest of us are.

A sad grey day of sleet and icy roads. Voting day. Well, I wore my Udall button, though I saw no other buttons of any political persuasion and found most of the people I spoke to weren't going to have time to vote.

March 3

Even worse than yesterday—I hope it's the last kick of winter. Sleet, freezing rain, travelers' warnings. And Udall came in second to Henry Jackson. But on the radio I have just heard that

Senator Stafford of Vermont has been directed (by what body I'm not clear) to introduce a clause stating belief in a Supreme Being as an amendment *to the Constitution*. That cheered me.

The priest came in handsome black and silver vestments to Mrs. R. and I suddenly realized it's Ash Wednesday. Presently he returned and gave her the ash mark on her forehead. I was most unappropriately signing my checks to send in to the bank. I felt like a money-changer, though this priest never gives me any feeling of the beauty of holiness.

One of the deprivations of this life, especially with a decaying memory, is that one can never look anything up. I am constantly finding that even my spelling is not to be relied on. It would be worse if one didn't care.

March 4

Low morale—reduced to crossword puzzle in the morning and stuck in it. This is partly congestion of the sinuses, which never moves; partly the winter landscape with nothing alive in it but two crows—twa corbies; partly Mrs. R.'s lingering illness and seeing her get weaker. Now they are going to move our constant neighbors, Mr. H. and Mr. O., who are part of our daily scene. Meanwhile Jessie, next door, keeps up an incessant shout. She says she has paralysis of the neck, but it comes out *paralys*—over and over she yells, "Girls, girls, paralys of the neck." What she has I don't know, but I still marvel at her vigor and volume. Mrs. R. still has the Ash Wednesday mark on her forehead and I find myself thinking, automatically almost, "Teach us to care and not to care"—which should be written up somewhere in all nursing homes. Now Jessie is crying, of her doctor, "He won't come, he won't come." She's probably right.

Letter from Jersey which made me cry with a desire to see my family—and no longer exactly homesickness. The occasion is the golden wedding of Tommy and Elsie on April 7 and I wished to be at the party they are giving somewhere near London for the family. In the midst of this self-indulgence, saw our long-time neighbors across the way moved here and there, shirts, shoes, radios, a plant, etc., packed on stretchers. One will miss the ritual conversations, most of all the good will.

March 5

Protestant service, with the comforting hymns again. Mr. Montgomery preached on the temptation in the wilderness, saying quite rightly that we are no longer tempted by the cities of the world—though one can have pangs. Only I can't follow him when he says we have the chance to prepare ourselves for glory. So many can prepare *themselves* for nothing.

Jessie again incessantly vocal. I believe Dr. Schwartz showed up for two minutes, but was gone long before she had said her say to him. So she kept on addressing him, long afterwards. "The first thing you've got to do, Dr. Schwartz, is to get me out of here. You've got to get this woman out of the room—she does nothing but talk in Lithuanian"—and so on. (As she says it, it is nearer *Lutheranion*.) Impossible to reproduce the effect, broken by cries of "Nurse" or bangings on the tray. Later I heard her say there was one nurse who was all over her, hugging and kissing her and she didn't like that kind of mushiness. She liked them to be sociable, which is asking a lot in one so antisocial. To my great surprise I found she'd once been a nurse.

March 6

This morning learned from *Country Life* that a new-hatched salmon is an *alvin*, then one of *fry* (does *fry* exist as a singular?), then *parr*, then *smolt*, all before it is a salmon. One has been caught in the Thames after 133 years, which also pleases me. But for the *alvins*, etc., I wish for a chance to use them, which will most certainly not occur and probably never has all my life. They will soon be forgotten in the swirling pool of lost words, lost facts, lost statistics—the pool images no doubt suggested by a picture of a fish-pass.

March 7

Sitting here, hoping to go home, had a visit from Mr. G. who had dragged himself all the way from the South Wing to see what seem to him like old friends. He says, "They don't care over there." Displaced persons.

This morning Dotty is more vocal than Jessie, and more like Martha Danielson in calling on names out of the past. This morning it was, I think, "Wilbur," with the refrain, which is the note of the place, "I can't get out."

March 8

A.J.'s Aunt Winnie died over the weekend and I found it hard to say to A.J. what I'd like her to know, as she shies off from emotion. The same day I had to write to C.—whom I hardly know, but have seen almost daily here—about her father whom I don't know at all, but who died suddenly at the age of 52. There there were no mixed feelings. It was like the death of John Russell so recently, leaving the family stricken.

The rest of my day has been heavy and lethargic, not much good to anyone. But I should record two good and utterly unexpected things. Kathleen made me a personal, hand-written anthology—she'd sent it by sea mail in January—a mixture of things from personal letters, to poems, to French carols. She mentioned she still had the French carol book I made her, copying them on music paper in the Leeds library that year I was out of work after college (a year that always makes me cringe when people say "they could find work if they wanted"). She said she had taught some of them to the children at school and I was touched. The other was an out-of-the-blue note from Cousin Bessie, as she signed herself, from whom I've not heard except about my father's death —twenty-some years ago—in all my adult life. She spoke of the happy times when we were "playmates" and I wept, remembering the Christmas Bessie appeared suddenly—her father brought her without a single thing for Christmas—and Mother rushed round and dressed a doll for her, just like mine with red cape and bonnet trimmed with white swansdown. I suppose I wept too because B. was nicer to my father than I was in the end.

March 9

A morning like Bedlam, chiefly Jessie, who has not stopped, and is even now talking to Mr. Drake after summoning him, the head supervisor and nurses in between. Mr. Drake is being very smooth, reassuring, tactful. She is going on talking to him, though he has gone. In between whiles she has demanded a wheelchair so that she can telephone her lawyer, her doctor—whose fault everything is ultimately—and her bank. I had thought she was *compos mentis* and just impossible as a person; now I am not sure. At one point all this was complicated by screams from Mrs. R. who still feels ill and for whom, therefore, every move of the nurse was wrong, and cries from Dotty. There is snow on the ground again. 4:30 P.M. Just at this moment Jessie is quiet. It is Dotty who is keeping it up and it is Alfred. "Come on, Alfred. Let's go. Let's get out of here" (repeated in various ways, though not very various). Then, "All right, goodbye. He's going. Don't go, Alfred," and, after much more, "I can't go now," as one realizes in a nightmare that all this isn't true, that one can't walk.

March 12

I ought to have recorded some of Jessie's ejaculations and conversations yesterday, when she had a spirited exchange with Jean, after crying out, "I want a top official." Jean said, "Who got you up and washed you and soaked your feet and gave you a suppository? Mr. Drake?" Today she was telling someone that the nurses lie and steal. But a little of her goes a long way. At the moment I feel unamused, as if I'd caught more cold going to the hairdresser and depressed at a forecast of snow.

Yesterday I wanted to copy down several things out of Giovene. But I read on—I finished Book I. The last chapter is very fine, with a poet's feeling for landscape, the seacoast and Ischia, where he lived in solitude, with casual contacts with a down-and-out peasant who was dying and with fishermen and a cat. Perhaps he is not really a novelist but essayist and poet. One knows his inner self without seeing him or hearing him talk. Some of his generalizations are many-faceted like a diamond. But many of his people—not his family—pass in a procession and fade. They don't say things one remembers like Tante Léonie or the Duke of Guermantes. (I suppose I think of Proust because of the many-volumed autobiography and the fusion of sense and intellect, but temperamentally they are oceans apart.)

March 13

More exhausted and cheerful. Read an account in a book of Elisabeth Kübler-Ross by a woman in a nursing home a little before her death. The end, with her acceptance of mere survival, was impressive (she was typing this a fortnight before her death) but she had not, for one, had to face—so far as one could tell—the worst horror, which is not death but senility. Her last words had still power. . . .

A day broken by visits; I visited Miss K., and called in on our late neighbors. Then another, who used to live next door, came down to see us and one had a feeling of warmth, though without the exchange of ideas. I get more of that with a few of the nurses.

March 15

On top of E. Kübler-Ross, read the obituary of L. E. Sissman. He was only 48. It must have been at the last Glascock Poetry Contest I was able to get up the stairs to that I met him, as I *think* I heard him read. (I am not sure about this.) I do remember he knew then that he had Hodgkin's disease and spoke of it quite openly. I think it must have been the last of the parties at our house. I'd like to read his poem called "Dying: An Introduction," written when he'd just learned he had it. I liked the bit the *Times* quoted:

> Tonight. Through my
> Invisible new veil
> Of finity, I see
> November's world—
> Low scud, slick street, three giggling girls—
> As, oddly not as somber
> As December,
> But as green
> As anything:
> As spring.

March 16

Serious snow, perhaps the worst storm of the winter. The radio at 3 P.M. is all cancellations—schools, colleges, churches. Six to twelve inches are predicted. I think of Elizabeth, snowed in, without Nora, and of her struggle later to get boys to shovel. I feel for all these hard-working people, setting out now, knowing they'll have to face much worse tomorrow. For me it is only a dark, grey afternoon with a fine, relentless snow coming down.

Have just heard Jessie say, to someone who went into her room and said, "I'm ———, I live here," "I don't want to know anyone here."

Mrs. R.'s misery is made worse by the fact that her son has not been to see her during her illness and this afternoon, as the nurse put her in bed she said, "Oh! Willy, Willy, Willy, Willy, Willy."

March 17

From an advertisement in the *New Yorker:* "The 1976 Impala and Caprice: full-size *sensibility* from Chevrolet" (italics mine).

A foot of snow last night, now driving in the wind, but with sun and not a cloud in the sky.

Jessie sends for the head nurse and says, "I'll tell you what is wrong with this place." It seems her principal complaint was that the nurses hugged and kissed her and this was not professional conduct. The head nurse replied, "Times have changed"—since Jessie was a nurse. I think how much they have changed from the old days in England, even when I was in Leeds Infirmary at 20; then no one could walk alongside the Matron to speak to her, and she gave a formalized, general greeting to each patient every day.

Went to the St. Patrick's Day musical entertainment, Irish songs and jigs, varied by "Ave Maria" and "The Blue Danube." The instrumentalists and singer not bad but it went on and on and the room got hotter and hotter until all I could think was, "I want to get out." The best thing was to see Mrs. R. swaying to the rhythm and beating time; the strangest—a woman who had brought her rosary, though she did not seem to me to tell the beads to any of the music, even "Ave Maria."

Heard of the death of Andrew Wood, the gentle gardener, who seemed so enviably able-bodied, raising his own squash and cucumbers and who in even cold weather, when the sun was out, wheeled his chair outside and sat down in it. I sat next to his crippled roommate, whom Andrew used to wheel about and take to things, who wept from time to time. But for Mr. Wood it was a good death.

Fascinating article in *Country Life* (by E. Lewis) on the old Welsh Christmas, with the children presenting apples stuck with sprigs of rosemary for their new pennies, and a horse's skull was brought round—that reminded me of my encounter as a child with the Old Tup, a sheep's head on a stick, which some boys brought in. I am sorry I was afraid of it and did not stop to hear the song of the last relic of mumming I'd ever encounter. She also mentioned a carol "All under the leaves, the leaves of life" which I'd like to be able to find.

March 19

Jessie is just saying she wants no part in all the card playing, beano, etc., that goes on here. "They chatter and fight and squabble. No sir, they aren't my people. They're not my people and I want no part in them." Now she's lost her footstool and is complaining that a thief came in in the night and took it. "Yes, sir. They steal around here. They've taken six pairs of socks and a dozen handkerchiefs and two pounds of butter." The question is, what was she doing with two pounds of butter and where did she keep it? I don't think anyone is in the room with her to listen to her bill of complaint.

Yesterday in a fit of recklessness ordered a dress.

Magnificent polemic against Nixon by A. Lewis in the March 15 *Times* (good old reliable Nixon) on the speeches since China: "That reassuringly familiar mixture of treacle and venom, whining self-justification and insult, moralizing and lawlessness, sheepish deference and lofty condescension. . . . One creepy touch of Nixon in the night and Scoop Jackson looks like King Harry at Harfleur." Good old reliable Anthony Lewis.

Another of the pieces Elizabeth sent out was a piece from Camus, a 1933 essay translated for the first time, which was full of things. I am not sure I see that "Freedom emerges from weariness," but on the matter of always setting out again, after a fall: "When some interest in our life crumbles beneath our feet, we transfer the interest we had accorded it to another possibility, and from this another, and again, without cease." And, "What does it truly matter what we lack, when what we have is not used up."

Effect of the impersonal voice announcing, "Activities are now over" while Mrs. R. yells, "I'm going to get so far out of here, I'll never come back"—that and much more, and Jessie yells next door for the head nurse and threatens to write to the trustees, etc. I can't help sitting and laughing to myself, then feeling guilty for laughing. One nurse had to cope with both at once, but she is young.

Last word: Jessie—"Get me a wheelchair to go to the office." Jimmy, in passing, "Take a cab. It's faster."

March 22

Dotty is now crying, "Mrs. Cranston, take me in, please," over and over. This is different from "Let me out," the common cry. It is sad, the child wandering in the streets, out in the cold. There was a time in my life, when I was still at Hood in the long-drawn-out depression, when I used to be haunted by the thought of being out in the streets when I was old, looking in at lit windows.

Home for a night—all good. Even the interview with Ovide Flannery over income tax was good—also brief—as I didn't have to pay anything and he thinks there is a good chance of my getting my estimated tax back. A few small crocuses, a nice clutch of snowdrops out. Inside lovely white tulips from A.J. Spent part of the time reading Elizabeth's manuscript. Arrived back to find Mrs. R. had been out for the day, but it was Irene, not Willy, who took her home. Jo gave me an old India paper concise Oxford dictionary—he said, "It's forty years old but that's just about right for us." Slept like the top I could never spin so that it slept. I used to divide people, for general competence, into those who could spin tops and those who couldn't. Who was it who used to divide people into Hamlets and Horatios—one of my friends? Christina? Myself? That would mean Horatio could spin tops as a child and Hamlet not. This is a game that would have appealed to Auden— the dividing, I mean, not top-spinning.

March 24

Kathleen's anthology, which she selected for me from her own commonplace books, had several things about age. But the one I am always coming back to is in the last chapter of the Gospel according to St. John: "Verily, verily, I say unto thee, When thou wast young, thou girdest thyself and walkedst whither thou woulds't: but when thou shalt be old, thou shalt stretch forth thy hands and another shall gird thee, and carry thee whither thou wouldst not."

In the state of happy expectancy—because it is a fine day and warmer—in which I feel someone *must* come to see me and still know I shan't be unduly cast down if no one comes. Read several of the poems of Seamus Heaney in the *N. Republic* and was much impressed. There was a comment by R. Fitzgerald, which I also enjoyed but am too lazy to get down to and grapple with. Laziness grows on one as routine becomes more acceptable. One asks, "Why should I?"

The expectancy was fulfilled. Two friends came, bearing hyacinths in pots from A.J. Even this room can be halfway transcended by hyacinths growing.

March 25

Enjoyed, with hot packs on my knees, an article in the *N.Y. Review* on James Merrill (by H. Vendler, whom I don't normally like very much). J.M. is one of the people I am glad I have met, who is kind, like Auden, and out of his immensely more complicated and brilliant gifts and the elegance of his life, could talk to us lesser beings in a perfectly direct and friendly fashion. I treasure a small compliment from him, as I do my larger one from Auden. I also value the long connection of the Glascock contest with J.M. from undergraduate on. There is a good deal in the review I'd like to copy down, but will content myself with what touches me most nearly: "If the divinity of youth was Eros, the divinity of middle age is Clio; if the metaphor for being thirty was embrace, the metaphor for being fifty is companionship; and if the presence in the mind was once love, it is now death." On Clio, I thought of Ben's essay on the weariness with criticism and the desire to work with facts. The metaphor for being 70, if it is a metaphor, is also companionship—I think it is *not* a metaphor in the sense that embrace may be. Death was not the presence in my mind at 50, as, naturally, it is now, but perhaps mutability was and a kind of exultation in survival. (I feel now, seeing Mrs. R. get weaker, as she eats less and less, that I am living with death—a long day's dying. Yet she can rouse herself to be angry, or to respond to company, especially male company.)

I feel I might be too lazy to read J.M.'s new long poem itself, except perhaps piecemeal. I will copy only "Already I take up / less emotional space than a snowdrop" and "What shall the heart learn that already knows / its place by water and its time by sun." Those two lines seem to me Elizabethan—except maybe "its place by water."

March 26

Well, they have taken Mrs. R. to the hospital, to my great relief—I think now she will survive. Yesterday I felt like Sir T. Browne in the "Letter to a Friend" that I saw the figure of death in her face and was alarmed at many small things: e.g., that she couldn't press the bell after I'd put it in her hand. She was in a daze—not there. Nor even angry. The head nurse says it is mainly dehydration and that they can soon get her over that, then get her back to eating again. But last night I heard one of the night nurses say, "I think she's dying." She has not talked for days, but still the room seems empty without her. All the same I feel a lightness and freedom as if I'd shed a skin—as if I'd been in hers.

March 27

Half listening to *Rosenkavalier* which is not my favorite, but very listenable-to. It's one I'd like to have seen in Vienna, just as I wanted to see—and did see—Mozart in Salzburg (but I'd like to see Mozart anywhere). I wanted to hear Verdi in Rome and didn't —managed only *Boris Godunov* and at La Scala couldn't get in to anything.

Thinking of Mrs. R. who, they say, is in about the same state as yesterday. It is the opinion of several people here that she has given up and does not want to be brought back. I feel as if it depends on how much her son goes to see her in the hospital.

I feel half guilty about having an orgy of public radio instead of station WHYN, which after all is a *good* popular music station.

A charming little Easter posy, made by our late neighbor's sister, whose name I still don't know. It is artificial but delicate, gauzy pink flowers and very convincing ferns in a miniature pink pot. And so kindly given. I do not even know her name and I doubt if she knows mine.

March 29

Seeing Mrs. R.'s things packed up in boxes and packing cases and knowing it is worse with her than they'd thought makes me feel I'll never see her again. They are vacuum-cleaning her closet. I think about a poem of Emily Dickinson—"There's been a death in the house" (probably misquoted)—where they throw a mattress out of a window—that always gave me the desolate feeling I have now. This was like a cleaning-up after a death, a routine affair which must happen over and over—also, of course, it happens when anyone goes home. But not many do.

March 30

The wandering Lithuanian, who does not come in here any more, has teamed up with another wanderer called Eileen. They go around offering help—and Christina, the Lithuanian, loves of all things to push the cart when they are clearing trays. Eileen, who looks normal, even well dressed, and speaks English, disconcerted me when she paused at the door, looking expectant. I said, "Good morning." She said, "No," then, "I really am telling the truth." This afternoon she disconcerted me even more by coming in and putting a pair of glasses down on my sink. I said, "Wouldn't it be better to take them to your room?" She said,

"Oh! I don't think you have to pay now." What kind of conversation takes place between her and Christina I can't guess.

March 31

Last night Mrs. R. died. I half expected to hear it this morning, having heard she'd had the last rites. I expected it before long in any case. I am surprised to find how much affected I am—it was the visit of the daughters-in-law and granddaughter that really upset me—the weeping women again. I have not been able to get Mrs. R. out of my mind all day. I was so used to her physical presence—her red robe, her flares of anger, her smile—rare since her illness. I thought, "Well, Anne, you got the hell out of here as you were always saying you would." I am afraid to think of what I may get instead.

April 1

IN MEMORIAM

Well, Anne, you got the hell out of here
As you threatened, not quite every day.
No need to walk out of the door in the snow
Or jump in the river. You crossed peacefully.
No more baths from these so-called nurses
(In this place calling itself a hospital)
Who scrubbed you as if you'd been tilling the fields
And shut off the bells when they wanted a smoke.
No more fretting over what you had once, what you had lost,
    what you had worked for,
The sandwich glass, the Haviland china.
Wherever you are, whether with Jesus, Mary, and Joseph,
Whom—Irish—you invoked in the extremity of
    exasperation
But believed in simply, firmly, as always;
Or whether you sleep in the *night of nothing,*
You are still in this room
A presence, more than a memory,
In your red robe like a Renaissance pope's,

With your un-Renaissance hair-ribbon, which did not
    counter
The hint, in some of your moods, of the Cumaean Sybil;
The deepset eyes no one would have known were blind
And the wide beautiful smile when things, meaning people,
Made you, a moment, happy,
Or when music played and you beat time
With your long fingers.

April 5

Waking depressed, after a weekend at home, I was cheered
by a letter from Susan, plus two other letters and a box of cards—
nice ones—from Mabel G.

I spoke to Jessie in the hall. She said, "How you stand walking up and down with one of those damned things I don't know."
Afterwards Karen, who cleans our rooms, said, "Just think of saying 'one of those damn things' to you, a college professor. It's like
saying it to the priest."

I am glad Susan is excited about the golden wedding. I feel
full of sentiment about it.

April 9

I should have said something of my new roommate earlier as
I've had her two days, but she hardly stopped talking long enough
to let me write anything. (I managed one very dull letter in bits.)
She is as far as possible from Mrs. R. except in her desire to get
out, but while Mrs. R. only threatened to walk out, this one put on
her fur coat over her elegant pajamas and, still in gold bedroom
slippers, got as far as the door, where she was stopped. (She arrived in a Cadillac and uses Chanel 5.) She reminds me of the
woman in T. S. Eliot—"my nerves are bad tonight"—whom I
can't quite quote but who wanted to rush out into the street with
her hair down. She suspects a conspiracy on the part of her husband and son and the good family doctor to put her here. No one
knows how she feels.

Later—already they've moved her. She has been moved where she can't so easily walk out. I do not know how responsible she is, yet she liked the programs on TV and radio which I had on and made intelligent comments on them. But when there is no subject from the outside world before her eyes, she talks exclusively of her symptoms, of the incompetence of the nurses, of the horror of nursing homes, where everyone knows you come to die. (Her father and mother both died here, but at an advanced age.) Her husband has just been to see me and she apparently had told him everyone here was a mental case but me. I liked him.

I was pleased also to have a visit from the sisters of the man who died back in the summer and about whom I wrote the not very good poem about their devoted watch outside his room.

April 14

This afternoon I get a new roommate. It is a beautiful day and Rachel, who once worked in the kitchen here, came in with daffodils—the nice small ones that look like the kind that grow in grass —or wild in Farndale, almost.

I do not know why I have been so lazy about writing things down. It is partly that some of the things have become routine— even Jessie's comments, which still go on next door, have become routine and sometimes like the cuckoo in July not heard. But sometimes Jimmy still makes me laugh as I eat my breakfast—e.g., when the rather fearsome Polish man in the end room was muttering in Polish what sounded like imprecations (but they can't all be) and Jimmy said, "That's just what *I* say." (*Muttering* is wrong —he was quite loud—*uttering* I suppose.)

Have now gone back to Vol. III of Giovene, the one I read first, and find it comes fresh in spite of the fact that I read it not much more than a year ago; now I understand all the references to the past. He annoyed me incidentally by calling Proust "debilitated and debilitating." Debilitated in a way, but throwing all his strength into his book. *Debilitating* I reject. "He gave me eyes, he gave me ears." I don't suppose Giovene found the Guermantes at all funny, having rejected that kind of society. He wants the meaning of life, Proust the essence of *his* life. They both say wonderful things about art. I am struck by what he says of the war in Italy (2nd World War) and how little the people had it at heart, how hollow they felt the Fascist exhortations to glory to be. It raises comparisons with Vietnam, especially the way people felt, in it and after, the last few years.

April 16

A heavy, lethargic day. Good Friday, as I tend to forget. My new roommate is saying a prayer. Coming down the hall with my walker, I passed Dotty who was saying, "The Lord will bless us all the same way. All the same way. The Lord will make us happy." Over and over—she is still saying it and from here I have just heard, "For ever and ever, Amen." It is the first time I have heard her not crying to be let out, or in.

April 19

Home for Easter in great heat, really sudden July heat which is bringing on everything far too fast, including the violets which have little short stems and look as if they'd like to be watered. I don't want spring to be over in a burst, with the tulips going up like rockets, and the apple blossoms out, then nipped. Everything at home good, though the sitting out had to be in the shade— friends, food, wine, a moving program on Buckley, in which we just heard Solzhenitzyn (sp?) interpreted, and then a discussion by M. Muggeridge and B. Levin with Buckley, none of them my favorite characters, but all moved and all talking about detente in terms of good and evil.

This morning I heard an old woman in one of the rooms (I persist in calling them all old women—she may have been 80) ask, "Does anyone speak Italian?", so I went in and tried my never good but now much diminished Italian on her. The trouble is I couldn't understand her except that she was from Napoli. I wish I could summon up a few of the commonest words even. I'm sure our conversation was all tangents and diagonals but nevertheless she blessed me and she had her rosary in her hand.

April 23

No one seems to be celebrating Shakespeare's birthday, but it is the Glascock Contest Day and that seems in the spirit.

Dotty is manipulating her wheelchair up and down the hall, without pausing for a moment in her monologue of distress. Just now, it is, "Rachel, where are you? I can't see you. Why don't you come? Rachel, I think I see part of you. Rachel, please. . . ." It seems impossible she should have the power to sustain it. Her voice is the last thing I hear at night. Last night it was as if they—whoever they are—were all going somewhere on an expedition. She was crying, "Hurry up, Papa. Come on. Hurry up, Grandpa." But you knew they weren't going to make it.

April 26

The reverend gentleman opposite (he is 88 and a Doctor of Divinity) talks loudly, almost sonorously to himself for long stretches. This morning when the therapist was trying to walk him, he stopped at our door and said, "You have a beautiful view, like a park." But then he went on, "If you had the money, you could build four houses there. But what is money? Metal." At this point Anabel led him away. At the moment, he seems even more inconsequent. When his roommate came in he said, "Are you bringing my supper?" And then, "Don't bring any donkey's heads in here" (curiously surrealistic). Earlier he was saying, "I've been here seven years (he's been here about two months) but now I've got to go downtown and work."

In the midst of this someone brought me an article on nursing homes and how some are enlivened by cocktail parties, dancing classes, patients being adopted by young people as their grandmothers, etc. I must say the effect was like a dead weight on the chest.

Home this weekend, chilly and rainy, but with the dogwood in full bloom and the Japanese quince—out before the orioles this year—and all the early shades of green all the way along the road, with shadbush, some apple blossom, all premature after the heat and charged with evanescence.

Today I want to do nothing but sleep.

April 27

Last night read Woodward and Bernstein's second book—
The Final Days or something like that—as excerpted in *News-
week.* In spite of the fact that it isn't and can't be as good as the
other—after all the other was their story, they were there—and
tends to fall back on the novelistic "thought Kissinger, reaching
for a drink," it is a convincing picture (to me) of a man who
couldn't see what everybody else saw. He is not tragic—the tragic
hero, even hero-villain, or whatever you call Faust or Macbeth,
must know. And I think Nixon still does not know, except that
everything went against him. But the spectacle of his refusing,
schoolboyishly, to quit—and all the other things he said about de-
serting the ship—while everybody, Haig, Pat Buchanan, even in
the end his sons-in-law, looked on sadly, seeing what he would
not see—is moving. I felt for Haig. I think Julie's and Tricia's refusing to believe it was a different matter. I think of the button
that was sold—"Nixon knew"—and of course he knew what he'd
done, but he never saw it as it was and what it meant and probably
never will. For the rest there were fascinating, and I am sure factual, details—e.g., that Ronald Ziegler wouldn't drink his morning
coffee except from a Lenox china cup with the Presidential seal.

I don't know why I have said nothing of my new roommate. I
am lucky to have her, so sane, good-natured, and accommodating. I shall not have her long. She prays for me.

April 29

I do not know why the decomposition of speech and reason
interests me, when it should appall me. I suppose because even
now I am interested in putting things together, knowing I walk a
narrow edge—that five, ten years, less, could disintegrate what remains of my power over words and logic. I am not sure what I gain
by putting down the forms it takes—does it amount to any more
than asking a few men in the street their opinion of this and that?
Nevertheless I was fascinated listening to Dotty in the interval between waking and breakfast, "Yes, sir, we'll all go tomorrow. We
can't go today. No sir, we can't go today. We'll go tomorrow."

140

Just like Gertrude Stein in—"Are two and two five or another question?" Since then I have heard a lot out of the Reverend Matthew opposite and his poor nurse has had a long hard struggle with him, getting him to have a bath, to go to the bathroom, etc., and meeting opposition all the way. I can't reproduce this and it was not memorable, except that I find no traces of the language of his profession in all he says—only the preacher's voice. He does not pray or call on God. At the end of the long labor of getting him up in his chair—and this, after all, in only one morning and one patient—I heard his Polish roommate say, as he went out of the door, "You were a preacher. You taught people. Now you old man and they tie you in a chair." A more effective use of language than anything I've heard out of the Rev. Matthew.

Later. As I walked down the hall the Rev. Matthew in his room alone was saying, "Rice pudding." As I came back he was saying, "Refrigeration." *Tout court.* Impenetrability.

May 1

Rain, so that I can regret less being here for the weekend. The grass, the trees, the freshness of everything takes the curse off. I am even enjoying the quiet and enjoyed reading a piece in *Country Life* on the ancient (Copper Age) monuments on Malta, with the mystery of their pierced monoliths and a perfect underground chamber. The lower half of a fertility goddess was visible in one place. It made me regret I'd not seen Malta—the very faint regret one has for all unvisited places (but how glad I am I can still feel Troy, with Dimitri reading aloud the scene of Hector's plume and Andromache, and the silence that fell on us all before we began to move about the ruins). The faint regret—the strength of one's present determination to make the knees move with the walker, but I am sure my knees are deteriorating and don't like to think of the ways I may deteriorate when there is nothing to rouse that determination.

But a good day, though with nothing to show for it. I almost got out the *Country Life* crossword puzzle, but as ever had two words wrong. I think there was one time I had only one.

May 2

A bad day after a good, as seems to be almost the rule. Too heavy for words and the knees sore when I tried to walk. Sat out and the day was beautiful, but sitting out in front, with constant arrivals and departures, a view of cars parked, though under trees, does not give me the pleasure I had last year outside this door facing the woods, with the chance of birds now and then. Was struck by the cheerfulness of the young man who has lost a leg and has some kind of muscular disease that affects his speech. "I enjoy every day," he said. Then came my Italian signora, all but crying, attended by a daughter-in-law and grandchildren but wanting Antonio, the son who had not come. "I want to die," she said. One of the grandchildren was pretty rude to her and afterwards I heard the two of them say, "She was a pain in the neck today." She is more *simpatica* in her room alone. But I felt depressed even before the arrival, and still feel I can't put two words together on paper. Thinking over the grandchildren, I realize I was not so rude, so *bold* with my grandmother, but was supremely uninterested in her and found it hard to see why her sons and daughters seemed to think her so wonderful. Recently I found out that Susan and Thomas felt somewhat the same.

May 7

A good day in spite of rain, though I didn't do much besides pay bills. Went to the Protestant service, which I found moving for the atmosphere rather than the words—though I was inclined to weep when Mr. M. said, "We come as sinners." And my sin is still pride, which takes all kinds of forms and sometimes tricks me by its metamorphoses. Reading E. Kübler-Ross on *Death and Dying*, in which I find the dialogues fascinating, I found myself thinking, "I'm not afraid of death," to remember I am afraid of decay, loneliness, loss of power and faculty, everything that goes to make up a lingering death. So all I mean is I'm not afraid of sudden death or cessation. And I go on indulging in minor personal vanities—e.g., I intend to send some poems out and find myself thinking, "They aren't so bad. They're better than ———'s." I am also pleased with myself that one of the nurses should bring me her daughter's source theme to criticize. But to return to what I am afraid of, I'm more afraid of Elizabeth's death than my own, or of a long or disabling illness for her. It seems the season for my friends to crack up—Connie is laid low, Jo dependent on drugs for his breathing and now Elizabeth has to go to the hospital for tests. I draw my strength and my supposed patience from them and the thought that I can still call 55 Hadley St. home.

There is a Spanish poem in one of the *Times* pages Elizabeth sent me. "Felicidad" by Jorge Guillen, "Felicidad es fiesta," but I'd better copy the translation as my Spanish (if it ever was mine) is too full of holes:

"Happiness" is a festival
"Happiness" would be too much
As a daily durable goal.
There are moments I feel fulfilled.
I don't call them "happy"
        I consume them
Leaving not a drop
        Consciousness
knows without superfluous fancy talk.
Let's play the minute with a mute
That'll temper our perfect harmony
If we can somehow manage it.

I especially don't like the translated line about fancy talk (Luis El-licott Yglesias) but feel a sense of recognition in the poem as a whole, except that when one is old one needs no instructions about playing the minute with a mute.

May 10

The Rev. Matthew in the room opposite is raising hell. The strength of his will is impressive as he stands there in the slightly ridiculous hospital nightgown with his thin legs sticking out. He is saying, "I won't be washed. I don't need washing. I want to get out of this building. I am authorized. I am insured," and much more interminably. Jimmy, Louisa, and Mrs. Baker were all needed to get him into his chair and tie him there. I cannot reproduce the inconsequent tirade that went on—it included duplicate keys and going to the hospital but he seemed indomitable and Mrs. Baker's "Now sit down and let's have no more of this non-sense" seemed inadequate. But how does one deal with immov-able will coupled with fluent—indeed nonstop—speech, to which there are no clues, except for the moments when he says, "I won't." It sounds as if it made more sense than Dotty's but that is only because it changes the subject oftener—it has more subject matter in fact but less connection, as Dotty's theme is always the same repeated. It is as if the others were always going off and leav-ing her behind—I see the train starting without her, or it may even be one of the old time wagonettes, like the ones my father's cricket team used to use when they played away, the ones I regarded as the height of bliss to ride in when they let me go along—the two horses, the men walking up the steep hills, and the hymn-singing coming home—"Beauteous scenes on earth appear," sung in har-mony, was the favorite. "But a better land by far / Is beyond / The evening star."

The Rev. Matthew is still chattering away to himself and, I take it, has not been washed.

What I want is a letter from my cousins.

May 11

In a way, the Rev. Matthew is the most depressing of all, not only because he is a D.D. and has had learning, but because he's left with the sense of authority he must have exercised and a sem-blance of the vocabulary—that is, no profanity, slang, or bad grammar—but without making sense. There's a song now that comes over Mrs. R.'s station, as I still call it, though I turn it on when it's Schoenberg or Messaien on my station—"Do you know where you're going to." No. No. Better not? I'm not sure. Mean-while I want to go and sit outside.

To return to the Rev. Matthew, because I hear so much of him (and now Jessie is gone, back to Amherst and the good soci-ety). He is reduced, because he must talk, to repeating words heard in the corridor, "O.K.... Between twelve and twelve-thirty. ... Can you help me?" and sometimes to the mere announcements over the intercom, "Mrs. Hill, call 58. Steve O'Connor, go to your office." In between, however, he has to say something—often it's calling for food. "A mutton chop would do." Indeed it would but it is a commodity unknown to these menus.

May 14

This month of May is going by without our being able to enjoy it. Cloud, showers, a fine day promised which clouded over. A poor April and a poor May. Elizabeth is in the hospital, having those disgusting tests. Connie is still limping after three weeks in bed. Paul is going to the hospital as an outpatient for tests. My friends are all cracking up. The Rev. Matthew has just announced he doesn't believe in suicide. It's against the law. "I regard it as murder. M-U-R-D-E-R." (And how far removed is proving to yourself that you can still spell from being pleased with yourself over getting a clue to a crossword puzzle?)

Most interesting review by G. Steiner of A. Powell's *Music of Time,* which he admires in a way which makes me wonder if I ought to try A.P. again. He ends with a quotation from T.S.E.:

All manner of thing shall be well
By the purification of the motive
In the ground of our beseeching.

This I believe, and can't achieve for myself, even here in this house of continual writing on the wall.

May 16

Stillness of Sunday morning. A blank in front of me now I'm up and swept and garnished. No poems to write. No letters I can write, though I've a long list I ought to write, because anything I'd write would put the recipient to sleep. And to think there will be a time when there is nothing but this, except perhaps pain.

My roommate reads prayers, while I read a life of Colette, thinking of all I haven't read and all I haven't felt. She was at the opposite pole from Giovene, whom I've just finished—not that his senses were not alive—in her immersion in the natural and her lack of arrogance. She makes me wish I were not so damn self-conscious.

May 17

A phenomenon of the Bicentennial has appeared here in a new hospital nightgown with '76 all over it in red and blue blendings. It is slightly absurd, like some other manifestations of the Bicentennial. One I approve of is the revival of canal boat rides at Windsor Locks—they had difficulty finding both a barge and a horse and there is some ridiculous red tape about their not being able to charge anything, so that the donor or organizing committee has to give it up after a month. I'd love to drift along at that pace for a while. (I sound as if I were going at express speed here.)

Nearing the end of *Death and Dying*, I am struck by the fact that most, perhaps all of the people she interviewed believed in a next world. I wish she'd had one infidel. Also I doubt that recording of other cases would help one much when one's own time came. I wonder. I believe it would help the people with families most.

May 18

Days like these, again marked by terrible lethargy, cut across outside by thunder and lightning, make one realize to the bone the meaning of "Desire shall fail." Desire is a shrinking circle, though there are still days when "The desire cometh" and "it is a tree of life."

Desire shrinks like a pond in summer (One will mind less when the pond's covered over, the scum unbroken. It is the agony now of knowing this and being powerless.) Water hyacinth—useless and graceless, grows over it. Soon it will be a pond on a village green, where the green scum spreads till it is like a floor. And the map of the world returns not to flat earth and the borders of undiscovery, but to the wall-map of the schoolroom, so many unvisited cities, lives, rivers without water, mountains—areas of dark brown. Till here and there, an old bonfire flames—we know for what it is worth, that I drank café in this most beautiful of all squares, that in a narrow street a green tree grew inside me as I said I am in Paris. A narrow street with a tavern at the end.

Lines for rivers where we did not believe in the water. Forests, marvelous patches of green and brown. The map returns—

but instead of "Here be cannibals," "Here I sat"—there in that
most beautiful of squares.

Areas of dark brown while we stared out of the windows
thinking of here and now.

Let others scramble for airports, lug bags. Now I think I have
committed the unvisited lands to the young and free. Let them
scramble—and like it—Till suddenly a home lights up.

May 19

The Rev. Matthew is on the worst tear yet. He sent two
nurses away—I suppose they were tying him up. One he called a
devil. "Get out of here, get out of here," he said in the tones that
must have echoed to the last corner of his N.Y. church. "This is
eviction from a private home." He still goes on—on fines, $1,000,
insurance, his wife. Still not God.

He has just said to a nurse who has gone in, "Don't talk to
me. I'm free."

A wet, wet day with hail, a few snowflakes and thunder.

Late flowers floated in a pool, when I just looked out then the
pool disappeared into a river. All the spaces in the woods are fill-
ing up with leaves, like water rising.

There in that most beautiful of squares I drank coffee like
nectar.

May 20

In bed last night thought of a dialogue between body and
soul, in which the body has the last word. It was the end of a dialogue—what can the soul say? It is the body triumphant, sure he'll
win, pointing out that the battle is already a losing one—that you
listen to music less, are less carried away by Bach and Mozart,
whatever you think you are going to be. That you look up more
than you are reading—"Who's that going past the door?" That
you are pleased with interruptions—a nurse coming in with pills?
You've come down on the world, down into the world, and what
a world—the small world of clocks and routines, wheelchairs and
commodes. You go to sleep when some CBS correspondent talks
from the wreck of Beirut. "Then soul live there upon the body's

loss," but you can't do it. "Soul clap its hands and sing?" How long since you clapped your hands?

Have finished the book on Colette, admiring her indomitableness, her energy fighting arthritis, her unselfconsciousness to the end, and envying the way she could sink herself in what the senses offered her—at the end fingering a shell, a fruit, or examining a butterfly's wings. I am sure I read a book of hers called *Pons de ma Fenêtre,* the *fenêtre* her last one in the Palais Royal, but I can't find it in the bibliography. There was a chapter on chestnuts, I remember.

Instead of letting myself get so preoccupied with the four last things, or one of them anyway, I should record the simple everyday things among the sane and the good—my roommate's sister praying to St. Anthony when I lost my scarves and then the scarves turning up, dropping down from somewhere when a friend put my coat away—after which I had Nancy light a candle for me to St. Anthony. Incidentally, the prayers in their Novena led me to St. Dymphna, who is new to me and who turns out to be the patron of the insane and mentally disturbed, a wonderful saint for nursing homes. I'd like to have the faith to pray to her this minute for the Rev. Matthew, who is asserting himself again, this time against the therapist: "I will not walk. I don't want you"; the unfailing kindness and patience of the nurses (not all at all times, of course, but most and most of the time) with those who are in need of St. Dymphna's ministrations—Eileen, with whom I've had inconsequent exchanges of words, whom they take with them when they're making beds or taking round drinks. She has been a nurse and likes to help. Kindness too of some visitors, e.g., one who came to have a picnic supper with her husband and found Christina, the Lithuanian, wandering in the hall and drew her in to the picnic. And for all there are the people who think their children have abandoned them here, there are so many daughters, husbands, sisters, who come every day, who have come to seem old friends and part of the scene. Then there is the young night nurse, 19 years old, who has to help care for a boy of 16, smashed and barely conscious, whom she's known all her life and who is being so admirable about it, though she cares so much—she is the one who made me read *Death and Dying.* And Miss K.'s humor over her being tied up as a result of trying to climb out of bed at night.

Even the very pleasant hot bath I had this morning when the nurse and I got so much involved in local history that I couldn't remember which parts of me I'd washed, and I learned among other things that Sophia Smith was a very jealous woman, who when her sister-in-law went in for white marble in her house, retaliated with pink marble (Margaret, the nurse, is an authority on the town of Hatfield) and the interesting fact that the town of Sunderland which was to have shared in Oliver Smith's charities got left out because some boys threw stones at his carriage. Early (or, on the other hand, late) vandalism.

May 24

Monday morning after a nice day and night at home, with sunny periods outside—few flowers except bridal wreath and still no orioles, but a pair of catbirds, a pair of cardinals and, most vocal of all, a wren who is leasing the bird house. Pleasant, wandering talk. Asparagus, which I've been longing for, not being resigned to insipidity—it hasn't even the distinction of austerity.

The Rev. Matthew is talking about hell, to which he has consigned Jimmy. It is the first time I've heard him on last things. There'll be a three-pronged fork, he says, that will "grip the flesh." I can't help thinking this is some view he held long ago, that he was scared with as a child, like the people who have terrified themselves with Foxc's *Book of Martyrs*.

This morning my station played Beethoven's little quartet—is it 13? (no, it is 11)—the second movement of which I especially love, especially the parts where the cello goes down and down alone. I learn that B. called it *Serioso*.

May 25

This grey May wears on. Today a pretty low point. Incredible meatloaf and canned string beans. I try in vain to encourage my soul to live upon the body's loss. Nothing in prospect. But last night had the unexpected pleasure of a visit from Elizabeth and A.J. in the course of which A.J. told me about a road she'd stumbled into in Virginia—a road which got narrower and at one point said ten miles an hour, where the birds got more and more as the road got narrower—thrashers and cardinals flying across the road, and a little flock of quail she had to stop for, finally a flock of grey geese. It seemed a kind of Paradise. It reminded me of those islands all of birds—were they Dutch painters who painted them? She must have felt she'd strayed out of the world.

May 26

Have just escaped from a musical entertainment, the worst ever. Al Ripley's orchestra so-called, and now known and to be avoided. There was an accordion, and somehow they couldn't control the sound and the microphones. Miss K. left before I did.

Thinking about the Liberal Arts—I think it was the Rev. Matthew started me, and the fact that he had lost Logic while retaining Grammar and the sound of Rhetoric, with some structure but without substance—I lost myself trying to reflect on their dependence on law. Arithmetic, Geometry, and Astronomy are so much more a matter of law waiting to be discovered. I suppose Logic and part of Grammar, also of Music, depends on law. But, as I said, I lose myself between art and science. All I can say is thank God for Grammar, Logic, and Rhetoric. And Music, of course, but not Al Ripley's "orchestra." (Logic seems to depend on a universal law whereas each race creates its own Grammar, but I suppose elements like tenses, genders and singular/plural are universal—or nearly so.)

Article in *Country Life* on a fascinating Armenian art collector who settled in Lisbon and left his collection to the city. (Was it not there when we spent our day there? Anyhow we never heard of it.) Some lovely things pictured. Why is one so fascinated by landscapes out of windows and why does one feel "If only I could get there?"

My no-longer-new roommate Marian took her first ride in a car and came back in a state of ecstasy. She has a wonderful warm spontaneous nature and I am lucky to be with her.

May 30

A Sunday I can't look forward to, with no possibility of a visitor and dampened by the thought of drizzle for Commencement and all the agony they'll go through about having it in or out. I put on a TV mass for Marian who decided to go and watch it elsewhere, so I looked at a little of it and disliked the jazz music, and undistinguished English of the liturgy and whatever translation of the Bible they were using. Also it seemed to me improper that the priest should begin by saying "Hello"—but I suppose it's a shade better than "Hi."

Have got hold of Colette's *Maison de Claudine* and am enjoying it. A very touching episode of the mother's first rather uncouth husband bringing her a pestle and mortar for a present and a cashmere shawl, having never given her anything, and I liked the picture of her calling to the children who were up trees or hiding in lofts in that place made for children.

I have now got Mozart's Requiem in place of that miserable stuff from Springfield.

I should record that yesterday the Rev. Matthew was quoting Corinthians on Faith, Hope, and Love. "Said to have been written by the Apostle Paul," he added, as if some scholarly doubts had come to the surface. It's the first time I've heard him quote the Scriptures.

May 31

Memorial Day, which means nothing much here, never did mean much to me in spite of the S. Hadley parade. Narcissistically I read through my May diary for last year, when I was still in hopes, though by then only half-hopes, of going home for good. I think I was more alive then, reacted to more things, had perhaps more interesting people to react to, but also worried more about money. Now I worry mainly about my knees—today they are very little use, though I've just had a painful walk. The housekeeping (there wouldn't be any today anyhow) has so broken down that dust stands thick on everything, unbelievable in this hygienic place. . . .

A nice thing while I was plodding wearily up the corridor. Ellen, whose young daughter worked here at the weekend, making beds, said her daughter came home full of thrill and said, "I used to wonder why you got so excited about the hospital. I thought it was just a job. But now I see it isn't."

I should record also, against my feeling of decline and fall, a few minutes of near bliss last night when I got in bed—and it's always a good feeling to stretch out my legs and let the bed bear my weight—and turned the radio on to the gaiety of Beethoven's third piano concerto. I was so elated I sang with it after my fashion.

Having complained that everybody says the same thing in the same way—I include myself, of course—I was surprised to hear the Rev. Matthew say, "Sex, S-E-X." Presently he was saying, "Winston Churchill. They called him the Grand Old Man."

Have just heard that the little Lithuanian died last night. She has been in bed the last fortnight and sometimes I've heard her crying in the night. She had rather a charming, elvish face and once took my face in her hands and said, "Peekaboo." I shall think of her working away with the broom, or pushing the cart with the dirty dishes, her hospital gown hanging down below her dressing gown, and a look of great seriousness about it, as if everything depended on her.

June 2

Today feel weighed down by the tears of things. My roommate is restless that things pile up at home and no doctor comes to see her and hasten the process of her getting there. Then we had a visit from Jack, the most pathetic of cases because he is all but dumb and can only make sounds and gestures and we can say nothing back. But yesterday there was comedy—we were visited in the night and wakened by a voice that said, "Hello folks. How are you? This is the Rev. Matthew Edwards"—but even before I could ring, a night nurse appeared. Then yesterday evening he got himself out of bed, where he'd retired early, and came out into the corridor in his nightgown with a plastic urinal and all his pads in one hand, and a pillow under his arm—intent and absurd. I don't know where it was he felt he had to go but he didn't get far.

After the lower depths of this morning, I had the best afternoon—here, that is—of the spring, sitting out on the lawn, new mown, with Elizabeth and Beatrice. An oriole was singing and one felt beyond contentment.

Good letters from both Kathleen and Louise. Louise meditates for about fifteen minutes each day. I can't, try as I will. It turns to undirected reverie. I suppose one needs a special kind of discipline I lack, though I could still discipline myself to read a poem. I should have been able to meditate this morning on what I was talking about in a letter, the simple faith of my roommate and her sister, compared with my failures. I do not get beyond tragedy and the knowledge that good is better than evil, though the bomb fall. . . . Actually, it is not surprising that one can lose oneself in a poem, which is an object—one gets inside it. The universe is too big. I remember being puzzled when Meribeth showed me a picture of an ancient stone head (of a Buddha? a Bodhisattva?) and said her friend used it as object of meditation. I am sure it is not like art, yet one wishes to penetrate inside something, into some heights or depths.

June 3

La Maison de Claudine continues to delight me by the vividness of recollections—things I couldn't recover however much I tried. Her father's political ambitions, his showing lantern slides to an indifferent audience, the horse's shadow—I can't recover any of the *sensation* of going with my father in a yellow taxi, where he was a Liberal Candidate for the West Riding County Council—only the words someone uttered when the rival got in— "What, has *that* mug got in?" And the air of pathos about her father made me think of the things we didn't want that my father brought home from auctions: stuffed birds, alpenstocks (which I liked), an aquarium with three fish which died slowly—as the stuffed birds moulted. And all those instructive books, Readers, once owned by Susannah Stevenson—one about children whose uncle would come in and say, "Let's have a chat about zinc." My mother called it "a lot of silly money" and probably dreaded his going to auctions. He never had any money sense all his life, though I was unaware of it until the age of 10. I suppose it was ultimately that which sent me to America—I felt as strongly as I ever felt anything that I must get away from his endless debts. I said, in intense self-absorption and with the sense of fighting for my life, "He's not going to ruin *my* life as he's ruined my mother's." But he didn't ruin hers. There was one day, when we were out walking at Brighton, she stood still in the street and said, "I don't envy anybody."

June 4

A fairly new, and very deaf, arrival. Frederick M. has just said what I've never heard said here before, "I'm so happy here." He said it in the loud voice of some deaf people, so that it sounded like a proclamation—or "Lift up your hearts."

June 5

Depressed in spite of lovely weather and two hours of enjoyment of perfect summer air. My knees work worse and worse.

The Rev. Matthew very difficult today and more than ever voluble. At one point he escaped and was found in the woods. At another he barred out his roommate, who had to force the door against him. In between he preached his endless sermon, or whatever it is—exhortation, conversation with an invisible companion, plaint, demand, echo. At one point I heard him say, "Don't bother with small sums. This is a big church." At another, "Cardinals, I never see them without thanking God I'm not of their color"—which recalls the Pharisee. Now he is calling at the top of his voice, "Supper, supper, supper." Once he said, "Twinkle, twinkle, little star."

June 8

Very nearly a day lost, uneasy and depressed. Disinclined for food. Dealings at cross purposes over a wheelchair I am trying to buy. Weariness with my own poems I'd been thinking better of, and weariness walking. The weather has changed to great heat outside, air-conditioning inside. At home on Sunday felt happy, especially listening to the Beaux Arts Trio—and watching it on TV —playing Schubert's Opus 99, one of my unfailing pleasures, which happens also to have been the first thing which made me know I was going to like chamber music. It always takes me back to the Robinsons and their civilized, unpretending way of life which introduced me to so many pleasures and took me out of my parents' quarrels for a while. I knew flowers and birds better for knowing that household, and food, and village life. And their old wind-up gramophone was my first real music, except for choir music and madrigals at college. And I admired M.V.R. for her elegant exclusion of what she was sure she did not want. On the other hand, yesterday in the campus restaurant, with so many familiar faces I did not especially want to see, in spite of being with friends I did, I felt the great gap between those who could walk and those who couldn't.

June 11

Horribly misanthropic, in spite of having acquired a wheelchair, having visitors, and, at last, having seen Dr. Brewster, who seemed to me—and I am sure this is common to patients in nursing homes—to dismiss me quickly and lightly.

Yesterday, on the other hand, I had warm feelings for my kind, when one of the volunteer men who come here to play cards and push people about told us about his wife in a nursing home, who did not know him, and about his own nine months at the Mass. General, in the course of which he'd been blind three months and his resolution on recovery to do volunteer work, especially for the old. Again I'm struck by the goodness and devotion I've seen here. . . . But I don't want Jimmy Carter for president.

The Savage God is very interesting to me quite apart from the spiral light on Sylvia Plath. The matter of tempting death, fencing with him, hoping to be rescued I find puzzling, though I'm willing to believe it. The historical summary was very useful—at least, I never thought of suicide as a crime and I'm not sure about people like the Samaritans interfering, except perhaps with the young. I had never realized either that Donne wrote "St. Lucie's Night" at about the same time as *Biothanatos,* I who once thought I knew something about Donne. (I was never more than half a scholar.) "I am every dead thing. . . ."

Fell asleep to the sound of Dotty's "Oh! dear, oh, dear" and "Mother where are you?" It is the sound of nights—if you wake it is still going on, though the robins are singing—as the Rev. Matthew's monologue is the sound of the day. Hers is plaintive, childlike, rhythmic, sometimes almost caressing, never angry. She speaks slowly, without a pause and has a range of notes. "Oh! dear, oh dear," is always low and full of regret. I listen and fall asleep again.

I am ashamed of my pin-head ambitions.

June 13

Return from a weekend to the sounds of the Northampton Bicentennial parade from the solarium, the sound of Dotty, still alone, still uttering her rhythmic cries—I thought of her last night when I woke at home in the quiet house and lay awake awhile, as I rarely do at home, pitying my aches, twitches, narrowing vistas, the wearing out without being ready to be thrown on the scrap heap. Then I thought of her, really alone as I believe, her people all out of this time—"Can you see me? I can't see you. Oh! dear. Oh dear." Mother, Grandpa, Arthur, William, Mary—and she inaccessible to the strangers in her present world. I thought, what nonsense to worry about rejection slips and nevertheless worried, or allowed my pride a small wound.

As against this, the perfection of the weather, the sitting out in strong summer breezes and warm sun, with all the leaves blowing, the poplar, as Jo said, sounding like a brook. The lushness of the heavy green of summer, a wren very active about his house, very loud and strong, a cardinal now and then, the "scissors bird" rasping away in the hedge or the wilderness. No "high midsummer pomp" but a few peonies, a few roses but fine ones, except for the hedge roses, half winter-killed, reverted to what they were once before they were grafted—like people still partly human after a stroke. Yet from a distance they made a show of white bloom. My vague malaise came from within, almost but not quite enough to make me wish, as I have wished before, that I could turn tree—I'd turn into our poplar today. But I still hope not tomorrow.

June 14

Today I'd rather not be a tree, partly because I'm trying to write a poem on Dotty, partly because at last I've had the letter from Susan that I wanted on the golden wedding, full of detail. The Rev. Matthew is so loquacious and so full of starts and changes. I can't keep up with him. As usual he is calling for Amy and spelling it. But he is also calling "Police!"—I think to untie him—and refusing his lunch again for fear of poison. Just now he said, "The town is surrounded," a moment ago he was calling the boys—whoever they are—to come right on in, "You'll get a message from the devil." "Come by the back door," he says. Perhaps there's a touch of Elizabethan there—Eliz. mad scenes, that is.

June 15

After his energetic, restless day the Rev. Matthew is silent and immobile today. They think he has had a stroke and have moved him where we shall not hear him—if he comes out of it. I hope he doesn't have to come back to the miserable remains of his life and the chaos in his mind, without any flashes of brilliance or nobility or even benevolence. Dotty's tiny circle at least is moved by family affection, a lesser star, however.

June 16

A visit from a brave woman called Jane Bradford, who told me without a trace of self-pity that they'd discovered she's full of cancer—"And so I suppose this is my last stopping place." She is cheerful, not to say spry. She makes me ashamed of my mood of yesterday.

June 18

My anniversary. I have lived here two years and survived, though not without scars and deterioration. (I was deteriorating before the accident, however.) This morning after hearing Elizabeth was coming out for a picnic and then getting the Academic Overture on the radio, I felt extraordinarily alive, while yesterday I felt shut in impenetrable gloom, changing only to a kind of desperation when I spilled a glass of milk over everything. I almost cried over the spilt milk—it was too much. A climax of absurdity and littleness.

I finished *The Savage God,* which I enjoyed to the end, though I can't say it changes my attitude to suicide in any way. It is full of things I didn't know, however—I didn't know what a poor, botched affair Cowper's attempt at suicide was. I know now too the difference between the real despair and nothingness of the world of the suicide and the passing darkness of those who play with the idea. He had a number of passages from others I wish I could copy. I'll copy one from Henry James (no source given): "Life is, in fact, a battle. Evil is insolent and strong; beauty enchanting but rare; goodness very apt to be weak; folly very apt to be defiant; wickedness to carry the day; imbeciles to be in great places, people of sense in small and mankind generally unhappy. But the world as it stands is no illusion, no phantasm, no evil dream of a night; we wake up to it again for ever and ever; we can neither forget it, nor deny it nor dispense with it." I thought *insolent* excellent. Later, returning the book to the nurse who lent it to me, I found she had copied the same passage.

June 21

Weekend at home clouded, as so much of life has been lately, by the weather—hot humid gloom. Have just been reading Hetsy's winter letter, with its long icicles and parapets of snow, and thinking how we longed for spring then and were more than half cheated of that by rain and that extraordinary burst of summer and now it seems we've been cheated of June too (there were three days of the real thing that I remember) by these hot lowering skies that one might expect in July. But my weekend was clouded also by a thick, insulated feeling (inside a lining, I felt), as if I couldn't rouse myself to be any use to anyone. The best bits were reading Russell Baker aloud in the *Times* and the Loch Ness monster, when someone else provided the wit. Also watching *The Lady Killers* and for the same reason. There is something ineffable about those improbable and diverse gangsters as a string quartet. I remember the last time I watched it, 1960 in Jersey at the *Omeroo* (was it?) Hotel with George and Susan. That was the very beginning of my troubles with my legs. Fifteen years and a half and they are still half-walking, at least bearing my weight. But to return to the weekend, I wish I were more fun for Elizabeth and not just a mass of demands, with my mouth open like a fledgling for what she can give me. And she gives and gives.

The longest day. I wish I could write about my feeling of its poignancy. Now the sun will be facing the wrong way. We've had half our light and what did we do with it?

June 23

Frederick M., the happy, deaf man who sits most of the day in the corridor, told his doctor, in the amplified tones everyone in the wing can hear, that this was the best place he'd ever been, that the food was wonderful, that he hoped nobody was going to kick him out. The Cooley Dickinson? He wouldn't go back there for anything. Doctors? He's getting along better without a doctor. I hope Dr. Smith found it funny.

June 24

Began very low, with asthma and melancholy. Wrote to Tommy and Elsie but found I was pitying myself. Surprise of a letter from Bernard de Reneport, after Bertile's gift of flowers, partly from me. He said the *jeune homme* of the picnic had become a *vieux monsieur*, father of two. I was touched to get it and admired the brief grace of the French. It was not only a touch of civilization, but a reminder of the day (very hot) when we went out on the Métro, with the basket and the wine bottle sticking out, like scores of others, and the graceful house we visited—Rambouillet, he said, but I'd forgotten. But it took an hour outside, even in the heat, to make me feel I could take things again. Only I'm still not sure I can.

June 29

Tried to lift myself by not very reliable bootstraps, out of gloom caused by all kinds of bodily malfunctions and minor distresses I find it impossible to write about, by sending a few more poems out, this time, merely doggedly, without hope—or with only as much hope as could get me through the process. Last night my roommate who reads me my Cancer fortune every night in bed advised me (or the expert did) to sell what I have, and all I have is minor poems. This coincided with the gift of a list of addresses from Louise, making it possible. It didn't seem possible to get outside—everyone too much occupied.

Am spending a few hours happily looking in St. Paul for a title for Elizabeth's book. She wants faith and works, but I believe she'll find more on building. St. Paul calls himself a master-builder, as Mary Lyon wouldn't have dreamed of doing, yet she willed her building into being, raised the money and counted the bricks made almost without straw.

July 5

End of the holiday weekend, which has had some of the best weather we've had, especially today. At home saw some of the tall ships, though we had to take a lot of parades, etc., in between the glimpses. One of the best bits was Walter Cronkite on the Danmark and the Eagle and the Danmark turning at the G. Washington Bridge. Apart from the ships, the best part was the bell ringing —I'd have liked more of what I think of as *real* bell ringing, but was delighted to find they had it in the Washington Cathedral. Among all the good things at home, including much talk, I want to mention the last two movements of the Mahler symphony on TV —Seiji Ozawa more than ever like that fawn with the archaic smile who haunted my childhood visits to the Leeds Grand Theatre—and also the little new beets we had with our good dinner, which seemed like the Tour d'Argent after most of my dinners.

Today I had a lovely afternoon outside (no need to get in for therapy, the other side of being deprived of it) and at supper a visit from Peter Remington. I am so glad he is coming to see us still after the death of his wife—the long slow death. He brings life and energy into a room at 80, knows and has known everybody and, as my roommate pointed out, never says a bad word about anyone. The extraordinary thing about him is that he still seems to get a boy's kick out of life, having known sorrow and loneliness enough. Even at his age, I wish he could find someone to marry him.

July 11

There are many things I've meant to put down, but laziness grows and I suppose the taking things for granted, as if this were the normal world. I read less, write less—though more, I suspect, than most people here—enjoy sitting out better than anything, in the shade of warm days with a breeze stirring, sounds of wood thrush and occasional cardinal, very occasionally the smell of pine.

Nevertheless there have been events this week. One was a select dinner for about thirty people, with steak and champagne. It was select, in that all the people there were *compos mentis*. It was an extraordinary mixture as regards clothes, however—some in hospital nightgowns, even in 1776 type—some in lacy, chiffony, old-lady type of things. I wore a cotton dress and my roommate something quite impressive from Angotti's. The food was good, so much above the standard that it's hardly worth comparing them, but the whole thing just missed being festive.

Another event was the arrival yesterday of the wedding party of my roommate's grandniece. The bride and bridesmaids very charming, also the bride's mother in a range of summery colors to match the day. Marian was bowled over by it. It was probably good for everyone to see them—so much youth and freshness, hope and flowers—their floating stuffs, garden party hats, and the perfection of summer weather, the kind every bride must desire.

A sad event was the departure of Jean, the nurse who has been here all the time I have, the one who lends me books and whose high spirits—singing and dancing in the halls—I have partly lived on. Yet she has no easy life.

Background to all this, the sounds from the next room, a Miss T. who calls out incessantly for everything, necessities and trifles, in a faint voice the nurses very rarely hear. "Oh! please come nurse. Louisa. Roger. Boys and girls. Oh! please help me"—then she cries, with the forced tears of a child wanting attention. Then her roommate joins in, "Crybaby," she says. "Get me out of here," says Miss T. over and over, and once a voice very much stronger than Miss T.'s, "Nurse. Come and get this woman off my neck."

July 13

My birthday, the third here and the saddest. The first, though I had to be lifted into the chair, was by far the most festive—champagne under the trees on a hot day and all the Reading Group and Jo sitting there, when I turned round at the bottom of the ramp and saw them. Then I had no doubt I'd get home, though I did not think it would be soon. The second was not strictly speaking here; I had it at home and the same people were there, but I got the cake and the Happy Birthday singing here the next day, to my surprise. Today was a day of cold, gloomy weather, no rain but no sun either—or just gleams now and then. I was still depressed from my visit to the dentist and the knowledge that the tooth that is bothering me can't be saved—and what is that going to lead to? But there was a very good letter from Susan, and one from Bertile with a charming French card of snowdrops—esperance, etc.—and a surprise one from Julia who re-created the prize-giving day at Wells Cathedral School most vividly—as she said, the essence or cliché of all summer prize-givings. Julia renews my youth, but not for long. Several people have told me I don't look 73 and I am glad of it, but Oh! God, today I feel it—73 and falling to pieces, knees, teeth, and insides. I wonder how Lord Clark, whom I still think of as Sir Kenneth, my exact twin at so great a distance, has passed his 73rd birthday?

The hospital gave me another hairbrush.

July 20

Next door those same two women are still scrapping, or rather one whines and the other scolds. I prefer the one who scolds and I fancy she is feeling ill a good deal of the time and the other's infantile crying and calling for Roger is the last straw. What will she do when Roger leaves—what will any of us do? Do without, as we did without Dick, I suppose.

I feel I should have so much to write, but the fire does not descend. Saturday was a good day, my real birthday party and Jo's, with a birthday cake and champagne and all the friends who have transported me (physically). I'd like to write a poem on champagne, but now feel miles away from it. Today weighed on me, even outside, except when I was writing to Muriel and had something to discuss. That is what one needs always, a subject, even if it's only Jimmy Carter—about whom we said surprisingly little, really, at the party, except to toast the Democratic Party's good health and agree that we'd had enough of little Amy.

And yet yesterday, when nothing happened and there was no approach to champagne, was a good day. It is only fair to say that. A hot but light dry air blew outdoors, as several of us crowded onto the back step for the afternoon, a row of wheelchairs and guardians. And I enjoyed very much Bellow's *Reflections* on Israel in the *New Yorker*. They gave me a more vivid sense of what it's like to be there than anything else I'd read. Everything precarious, warm, salty, intellectual, contentious, in the midst of the perils we see far off every night under the aegis of Walter Cronkite. Good on the idea that democracy depends on self-discipline, and that— as a consequence?—periods of real democracy have been brief. "Our species knows little about being free. Ruskin writing of Thucydides' 'History' says that his subject was, 'the central tragedy of all the world, the suicide of Greece.' " (Where does R. say this?) That reminds me that yesterday I also got a letter from Hetsy, very evocative—she still should write a novel—in which she offered me balm to the spirit in admiring my poem, written in the heat of the first reading, years ago, of Thucydides, and told me her son was moved by it. She is another of the blessings I should count, and not for such crumbs of comfort either, but that I knew her, "had" her, as we say of students, and know her now.

July 25

July wearing away. Yesterday at home a good, though quiet day. No company—just talk and reading *The Book of Abigail and John* and watching Buckley argue with J. K. Galbraith. Today less good, because I was off my food, not because of the day which was perfect though I couldn't rise to it. Came back depressed by Elizabeth's health, by mine. By the fact that the garden gets out of hand for her as well as everything else. That it can't last, can't last. "What to make of a diminished thing."

A visit from Peter Remington, whose wife died so recently, he armed with a notebook from which he read me—reflections on the laundromat, the seasons, a story his wife wrote for her kindergarten class. I was touched (though distracted because I wanted to get in my walker and can't since my mechanized chair broke down). He said it sometimes came upon him after he'd got into bed, the desire to write, and I thought of all the degrees of "inspiration" and that led me to the "absolute poem at the center of things" (probably misquoted), the reflections caught from reflections and how we all have our moments of feeling it's the real thing.

AN ANSWER TO THESEUS

Not out of airy nothing, Theseus, he made this play.
Take the moon—and Moon is a principal, without him no
    play—
That was made of moons from the beginning:
Nights of light in flood over river meadows
(Good hay, sweet hay, with haycocks for lovers)
When trees in a park sailed free on their shadows
And the deer slept; nights of cloud-curtain and
Sudden appearances, working their trickeries
Even on the cottage where the plowman snored,
Raising ghosts in the churchyard—on such a night,
Lated in a wood, a man might thrash through
Cobwebs, tangle in bush and briar, to emerge on
Clear spaces, dancing floors, every fret of a fern visible.
Times afterwards at my lord's, when the moon peered in
Through the Great Chamber window on players in motley,
Or on the Bankside stood above spires and rooftops,
Local habitations, innyards tilting under feet going home.
No, it was out of the moon from the beginning,
With all its charms, influences, gods, powers,
And the man in it, even his dog, he made this moon
Which confounded the calendar, still shining
As it shone that night, very constantly all that night
Till your hounds, Theseus, flicked the dew away.

July 26

A much better day, with an ideal temperature outside in the afternoon and an hour of pleasant solitude which fell short of a "green thought in a green shade" because there was hardly any thought, also a small bit of guilt at staying away from a big gathering at the front of the house with punch, etc. I shall never reconcile the feelings of "Why shouldn't I lead my own life here?" and "Someone has taken a lot of trouble to get us all together, therefore I ought to go." Meantime I enjoyed the ferns and pine.

Pathetic—absurd episode of Miss T., the crybaby from next door, outside our door where she had somehow got herself, tied in a wheelchair, but couldn't get herself back. She circles with one hand on a wheel, the other on a brake, asking everyone to take her dress off. When I finally got someone to wheel her home, she said, "I have such a hard time."

August 3

Cheered by the *Sunday Times* excerpt from Elizabeth's (my cousin's) book on her farm with a very nice almost full-page picture in color of E., Desmond, Rachel, and some charming kittens, a dog, the farm mostly hidden by trees in the background. I hope the book is a great success. This arrived as I was working on the highly improbable job (for me) of going over the English in Anna Jane's chemistry notes—intended for a text, I think—which she will hand out to her students. The moment she got into formulae and models I was lost and can't always tell whether the English is good or bad, but I am pleased to be doing something which I hope is useful, though I can't be certain.

Warmed also to receive another check from Thomas, which more than counteracts my bill for teeth from Dr. Vassar Higgins. But I must tell him to stop sending me money till I really am a pauper, not just beginning the downward slide into penury.

Reading a review of a life of B. F. Skinner, autobiography in fact, was interested that he'd wanted to be a writer, had certain gifts and some success, but lacked something—the essential—and so turned on art as something meretricious, ruling out even the great—e.g., Proust—as if they were just on the wrong lines. It explains the gap between us and the Psychology Dept. It is as if there were only one way of looking at life, as if I ruled out Anna Jane's chemical formulae and ball and stick models.

August 5

Worry about Elizabeth in hospital and how much they can do for her, how serious it is, how long she can carry the burden of the house—last weekend I saw the leaves closing in on her on all sides. Worry about my roommate, who goes on having an undiagnosed pain in her side without any help or even interest from her doctor, and the effect it is having on her spirits.

In spite of which I enjoy the time outside and have all this week of sun and not too high temperatures, with warm breezes and always the smell of mown grass. This summer I sit with a company of widows or spinsters and one happily married woman of 86, who has bone cancer. A change from my old benchers of last year, the gentle Mr. O. whom I hardly see these days, Mr. H. whom I see often in the distance and hail, though he can't hear and Mr. W., now dead, telling one with tears that losing a wife was losing everything. Also Mr. T., with his air of the world.

Frederick M., deaf and happy, has a childlike innocence and ingenuousness as he shouts his opinions for all to hear. He has just been talking to the new young man, Harry, about the incomparable Roger, now driving out to Minnesota. (This is Missing Roger Week.) He said, "It makes me think of Lindbergh setting out across the Atlantic, with all its hazards. There's Roger setting out with all the hazards of the road. I hope the poor young man makes it." I think R. would be amused. "Did you ever meet Roger?" Frederick asks Harry and Harry, who had not, is probably going to be tired of hearing the name of Roger.

August 6

(Susan's eightieth birthday.) A letter from Kathleen, with the remark, "Isn't it a good thing one doesn't realize at the time that one is doing something for the last time! Do you remember when you last walked off a tennis court? I don't." I don't think I do, but fancy it was at the Robinsons', at Swarraton. When, I don't know. I am sure my last swim was off a Greek island, but couldn't say which—or perhaps it was in the Hellespont or near it, when we didn't go to look at the war memorial to those who fell in that region in World War I. I think my last really happy swim was at Rhodes on the first Greek cruise. That was a perfect day. As to the last time I *enjoyed* walking, it was Christmas 1960, after the long period of sciatica in Jersey and the first weeks of Wm. Goodenough House, then the British Museum seemed too far. But we walked up the hill at Caterham to where the view is, on a lovely, mild Christmas Day, and I felt pleasure in the use of my legs again. Not for long.

August 11

Writing to Elizabeth in hospital has been the chief reason for writing nothing here. Also I have put in a fair amount of time on Anna Jane's ms, from which I must put on record the fact that an *inert* gas is also called a *noble* gas. I must inquire into this. Another sentence that opened up possibilities was: "Every electron repels every other electron and a nucleus repels all nuclei, but an electron attracts all nuclei and a nucleus attracts all electrons." I feel there ought to be a novel or a play there. *Couples.*

A lovely afternoon outside, watching men work—mostly one man, the good maintenance man who took my chair to be mended —stripped to the waist and brown as a haymaker—clearing away the oaks that had been cut down. Smell of new-sawn wood, bundles of foliage dragged and lifted by a tractor, then logs loaded onto a truck. I think the trees, which were half-rotten, were cut today because of the threat of the hurricane two days ago. They were not beautiful, but I shall miss them. Mr. D. had counted the rings and they were 69 years old.

We have another wanderer, a much more vigorous one than the Lithuanian. I am astonished by the vigor of this woman, in fact, and her appearance of health, but she has no idea where she is and is always straying into other people's rooms, sometimes taking some of their belongings with her (she took a shirt and tie pin from the man opposite). The night the hurricane was supposed to come, she raised hell, getting out of bed repeatedly and

167

fighting the night nurses who tried to put her back to bed, until they got a young man to come from another wing and tie her down in bed. I heard her say, "I'll break your glasses for you." One nurse said, "I guess we had our own hurricane." Last night about 2 A.M. she was in our room, but just sat down quietly and permitted herself to be led away. There was a comic conversation between her and the deaf man one morning, he hearing very little, she taking off from various things he said into private memories. At one point he told her a man's best friend was his mother—he'd taken care of his till she was 97. "Except God," he went on to say. She said, "You're not kidding." After that they sang "God bless America" in something like unison.

August 15

This is the 89th birthday of the deaf man, Frederick M., and no child could be happier about it. It is wonderful to hear—and of course we hear it—such joyous acceptance is much too passive a word for the way he meets life. Everyone is so good. "Thank you, nurse. You are so kind." Every morning when he wakes he thanks God that he is here. One feels he will go up to heaven with a great shout.

On the other hand, there is a new woman next door who screams if anyone goes near her and pushed her tray onto the bed this morning, purely in a fret, as far as I can make out.

Somewhat rejuvenated by a visit from the Ellises on the crest of a wave, after grandeur of an eighteenth-century house in Bucks last year with grounds laid out by Capability Brown. Nadine came with them and talking theater again—I'd really given up even thinking about the theater—I took pleasure in remembering old performances, and the Malvern Festival years, with the incidental pleasure of coffee on the terrace and the possibility of seeing some of the actors, the kind of possessiveness one develops seeing the same people often—we had it with Pierrots, cricketers, even later on with people we saw from year to year like the musicians at Marlboro. I once wanted to write a novel with the Malvern Festival as scene and climax. It was to be called *Interesting People,* I remember—my heroine, Griselda, had a crush on an actor, but married an ordinary young man and decided all people were interesting. I remember Meribeth saying to me, drily, when I told her the conclusion of my plot/theme, "I can't agree with you there." And I never got beyond Chapter I.

August 19

There should have been so many things to put down these last few days, if I hadn't been writing to Elizabeth every day and finishing A.J.'s ms, the carnival, Elizabeth's (Cragoe) book, the death at last of Dotty. I went to the carnival partly to see what the word meant in an old people's home, though I'd been warned to put all ideas of Mardi Gras out of my mind. There was a clown, i.e., a boy (I think) made up as a clown, but he did not go in for any antics that I saw. He was just there. There were stalls, with darts, rings, etc., where one might collect tickets and so perhaps win a prize. I tried only the fortuneteller, who was a night nurse effectively made up as a gypsy. She told me what she thought I'd like to hear. There were balloons on strings. There were also hot dogs for those who waited for them. But out of a beautiful week, they had chanced on the only cloudy day with a cold wind and I did not stay long. The best thing was a fife and drum corps from Easthampton made up of what looked like cub scouts, junior high school girls and a mother or two, or perhaps one was the band teacher from the Junior H.S. The six young girls playing "The Minstrel Boy" on the flute were quite moving. And the tiny, highly miscellaneous group had excellent seriousness and rhythm—also some handsome banners. I felt they were worth the price.

Heard of the death of Willy, Mrs. R.'s son, whom she loved. One can only be glad that she died first and that he did not go on living any longer as he was, destroying himself. There was something warm and generous about him, but evidently his alcoholism was incurable. I think of the cups of tea he brought me from "Dunkin Donuts," black and stewed so that I could hardly get them down, and the dandyism, the delight in his new shirts and jackets he had to show off and the way he changed his mother's face so that the light came into her eyes and she looked twenty years younger, and her sad belief in him—"I called Willy and ten minutes later the power came on." His wife loved him too and must have suffered these last months. I'd like to write to her, but feel there is nothing I can say.

Elizabeth Cragoe's book: I admire a good deal about it and shall be interested to see reviews, if I do see them. To begin with it is highly readable, lively and unselfconscious—I could never at any time have achieved that degree of unsentimental ease in talking about myself without some element of disguise. I think she has excellent powers of organization and exposition—I personally enjoy being told the facts of haymaking, etc.—with a very nice sense of what a paragraph is. Sometimes too, especially in the flower parts, there is a very nice sensibility—e.g., she has really looked at a celandine and made me see it. Naturally, I am a sucker for all the wandering in lanes between flowery hedgerows or calling the cattle home—full of nostalgia and what will never be again and all the pastoral poets. I am overcome by all their sheer hard work, shoveling muck, baling hay, etc. Desmond Cragoe, whom I scarcely knew before, emerges in quite a new, heroic light. The book is built on their effort.

As to Dotty, we shall not hear her voice any more in the night, but no one could have wished her to live on.

For once the *Mt. H. Alumnae Quarterly* was full of interest: Susan Shwartz taking to pieces Elaine Becker Kendall on *Peculiar Institutions;* a few student papers, one of which on Lilith and Blodenwedd, a Welsh Eve or something like it (she didn't say whether B. was the first woman), I found really interesting. Blodenwedd, however, was made of flowers, and at first nonhuman. When she did become human she turned into someone more like Lilith than Eve, though I have to admit I'm not reliable on Lilith, less on Blodenwedd.

August 22

I wanted to copy "Thucydides" as I keep finding myself without one. Am sending out a few more poems, without much hope, yet with some or I would not do it.

Still, I want to send this one out and it's all I have.

Summer was now over:
The trophy set up for victory,
The dead all buried; and now there were ships
To be hauled up and caulked in some foreign port,
Hulls careened, ropes mended,
Walls put together stone on stone or sometimes taken apart,
Slowly to the slow file of images through memories,
For every man his own but for all smoke rising
Across waves like mountains between the mountains
Of hibernating islands.

Summer was now over, but now
There were envoys to be sent, words, words, words:
Sides changed, weight shifted like freight;
Prices fixed in the market (What is today's price
For slings, oars, skins? What price honor in the agora?)
And promises fretted away like bad cable.

Summer came back over and over,
Lean and tanned to the arms of the hard country,
Bringing the wine and the black shadow of leaves to the
         marriage feast
And passed with the last dust of fragrance from basil and
         fennel.
But he, writing his history in stainless daylight
Saw beyond hope
That one high summer was over for ever;
Stopped writing and looked away,
As once Zeus turned his eyes away from Troy.

It seems strange a whole morning could go in sending poems to
two places—much of it, of course, consisted of trying to get hold
of the envelopes with the poems in, dropping them on the floor,
trying to sweep them toward me with a pen or the legs of my walker. (My roommate is always dropping her prayers on the floor and
in general specializes in losing things and looking for them.)

The afternoon was utterly idle, except that I learned from a
New Yorker item that the people of Frinli speak something nearer

medieval Latin than Italian—their days of the week are—*lunis, martars, miercus, ioibe, vinars, sabide,* and *domenie.* This piece of information occurred in a really moving account of the earthquake in a town in Frinli, when the narrator's first thought was that they'd been hit by an atomic bomb. How strange that the Act of God had come to be the second thought, not the first, and what a comment on our precarious footing in these years.

August 25

A momentous day for Marian, my roommate, as she has been told she can go home tomorrow. The shock of it reduced us both to tears. In rejoicing with them that rejoice, of course I can't help asking, "What now?" And just at the time when I can't go home. It sweeps over one again—I can't get out.

This morning we were laughing over the murder mystery set here—the corpse obvious, the motives so manifold that anyone could be guilty—that could be written, and that they wanted me to write. (Only I can't, and never could have. My idea would have been to import Virginia Ellis as a disguised volunteer something-or-other, and let her talk to all ranks and departments.) But someone who knows nursing inside out should write it really. This morning too, I felt activist about the want of help, the want of supplies—blue-pads withheld, towels with holes in them, etc.— enough to consider writing both to Conte and his opponent in the congressional race. Well, I am thankful I can still have such a wave of energy—now I only hear its melancholy long, withdrawing roar. Only I'll get over it, recognizing I'll feel so less often, that Elizabeth will feel so less often—that my next six weeks here will be a dividing line. Also that summer will soon be over.

August 26

Marian gone with tears. The room in a litter. A feeling of desolation and loss and also that one's world will be made up more and more of the passing and temporary. That this will substitute itself almost without my noticing for the semi-permanence of S. Hadley, that conversation will stay in the shallows until perhaps there will be no depths to get down to. Except for loss. Sad letter from Rome in the *New Yorker* about politics, but also litter and squalor in the Piazza Navona and Piazza di Spagna and refuse and roaming gangs of boys in the Forum.

August 28

Terrible oppression and feeling that all is vanity and vexation of spirit, that I can't make myself write to anyone or write for myself. My new roommate is very nice, very accommodating, very simple, and makes me ashamed of myself. My roommate thinks I am a nice lady, which I am not.

August 29

Third day of this apathy and the black dog on my back and today there is no consolation outside. Chill and damp with, now, pouring rain and a feeling that the future will be like this, that nothing can get through to me.

P.S. The future stopped being like that no later than 2 P.M. when Elizabeth and Bea appeared and we had a nice hour out on the doorstep. There is nothing like talking to people one knows about people we all know. But I see that it will be a long time before I can go home.

September 4

Of all things I have just heard over *Morning Pro Musica* (under the title of Sentimental Songs of the Mid-Nineteenth Century) "Father, dear Father, come home with me now" and "The Grandfather's Clock." "Father, dear Father," especially seems to belong to my early years, when the "drunken man" was a kind of bogey in our lives and the rows of men "cronking" outside the Halfway House at Robin Hood, waiting for opening time, was a familiar spectacle, when we got off the train there. "The clock in the stable strikes one"—I wonder how many stable clocks there are these days?

I ought to have broken through my lethargy and pure dullness to record the excitement of Thursday afternoon when I became for the moment involved in the politics of the place. For the first time I see what County Commissioners can mean in my life and the whole life of the hospital. I felt at the time I'd like to go round distributing handbills saying "Vote for Garvey." It is not only that Garvey turns out to be married to a former student I like, but that he came here to see what it was all about and talked not only to our manager, who did not at all like his talking to the nurses and patients. Even the Director of Nursing said to me, "If ever you write that book, tell it like it is"—Charles, the solid and invaluable, who has been here 25 years, told him we were kept short of soap, linen, etc. He also said, "If you get elected, don't just talk in the office, talk to the employees and the patients." Everyone was all agog and I wished I could do more than put in an application for an absentee ballot.

September 5

Labor Day—a perfectly beautiful day, with a clear sky, warm sun, and a cool wind that felt exhilarating, as if it came from the sea. After sitting out morning and afternoon, I felt drugged with air as if I'd spent a day at the sea—I was reminded of Labor Days I'd spent in Maine, with the dew on the blackberries, and one in particular when Elizabeth and I picnicked on a rock near Blue Hill, then went to Blue Hill Fair where we saw charming Alpine goats. The climax of yesterday was that Elizabeth came out, brought by Bea, and we sat in the sun—I hope they felt the sense of content I felt. It made up for our fiasco of a picnic on Saturday, when the weather turned cold and bleak and the thermos fell on the floor and broke before we'd had any tea. One sad thing, the Harvard Press had rejected Elizabeth's book and I was ashamed of being cast down over my paltry rejection slips—after all, my poetry, such as it was, is really over. Her book is the solid work of several years, and the close struggle with hand-written letters in the heat and cold of the Archives Room and she knows more about Mary Lyon than anyone else in the world.

September 12

So much good and bad I don't put down in these autumnal days, when one rushes (not the word for me) outside to seize any

174

gleam of sun and custom lies upon us like a weight, etc. Frederick M. goes on booming to the world how happy he is, what a wonderful pineapple he has made in Crafts—now he is working on a rooster—and Peter C. next door goes on thinking of him as a damn fool. He, Peter C., is sad and restless, trying to get used to a new leg and finding it painful, not sleeping, not knowing where he'll go when he is used to his new leg, alone with only a son in California. He is both patient and impatient with the tiresome, querulous woman next door who still cries for attention and gets herself in a wheelchair outside his door, calling "Peter, Peter." After a while he comes, and shows her many times over that one can't move a wheelchair with the brakes on. I was glad the nurses took him to the County Fair.

A terribly sad case just moved in—and to Jane's room, when she has already so much trouble of her own and her husband's. This is a young girl with Huntington's chorea—in her twenties with an eight-year-old daughter. Her husband has divorced her. She lies there, all convulsive movement, hardly articulate at all. What can one say, except to hope it will not last long. I wonder how E. Kübler-Ross would deal with such a case? I wonder what is the future of the eight-year-old girl? If I could pray—and I have just watched the same uninspiring mass on TV—I would pray that all those without hope might die, that Jane's husband might not have to linger—she hopes this too. Lucetta, whom I passed when I was walking, was crying because her knees hurt, her TV wasn't working, her son didn't care, but said, "What can you do but pray to the Good Lord and our Blessed Lady?" But I keep coming back to the girl of eight, and the hereditary disease.

I should put down my letter from Sister Estelle Moriarty, one of the daughters in my vigil poem. (The two sisters came in to see me and I showed it to them.) I decided that perhaps this is my audience and the substitute for publication. My first letter from a nun, who said she was proud to have been part of the vigil, and that God would inspire me. I wonder. I seem to have grown a thicker skin since then.

September 17

Low point, a mixture of the grey weather and steady rain with steps taken to sell my dividend shares to keep me alive in a place where I do not wish to be (there are much, much worse). Plodding the corridor, I thought of my feeling one day as I looked out of a window (and I think it was in Texas) and thought that the fountain of youth remains constant on any campus—the young girls on their way to class are always the same age, while their guardians get older, though youth even then is always coming in. Here there is still youth and it keeps us alive. I like to hear the young nurses singing and whistling in the corridors—it would have shocked Florence Nightingale. They give us their life's blood. Well, I suppose that was what we gave to the students, and what parents give. Only it seems we have little to give these nurses in return.

September 23

My third roommate departed, happy, for Easthampton (my fourth if one has to count the one who stayed two days and wore a mink coat). I am afraid I harbored thoughts I'd like to be able to take back now. I felt she wanted more of a response, more of a demonstration of affection than I could give. Once she said, "Joyce, don't you ever wish you was home in your own apartment?" and I wanted to hit her, or on the other hand, burst into tears. She told me the same things over and over. (This will happen to us all and I know it. It has probably already happened to me more than I realize.) . . . I have just heard the Signora up the hall ask, "Have we had breakfast?" It is 5 p.m. and we are waiting for supper.

My new roommate, 90, rational and, so far, querulous, did not want to be moved and still resents it. She was said to want conversation, which I think a misinterpretation as she has several times said she wants a private room, and to like music, which I don't believe as she puts on a station considerably lower on the scale than WHYN. I foresee difficulties and must try to cultivate the shell of the turtle—I already have his pace.

Everyone is stirred up because there has been another fit of moving out the relatively able-bodied—I find they are grade four patients. I think I am grade three. I toy with a short Op. Ed. piece for the *Times* about the plight of those in nursing homes, those wanting to get in, to be of the same grade as their husbands (Jane's problem—she is here and her husband in a so-called rest home in Easthampton), those put out.

They have just moved my latest roommate back. She made it so very plain she did not want to be here. Now what?

September 26

Have just listened to Rosalynn Carter on TV. She is a sweet thing and a confident enough speaker, though with a small vocabulary and a small stack of ideas (I am reminded of what Peter C. said about Mrs. F., though she, "unlike most people," as he so justly remarks, suited the number of her words to the number of her ideas). I wonder if she can be as unsophisticated as she appears? Probably not, after all her campaigning. The funny thing was the presence of George Will on the panel, looking as if he wished to be disassociated from the whole thing. They asked her if she'd ever seen *Playboy* (to which Jimmy had just given a notorious interview), and she said, "No. But 40 million Americans read it." Perhaps the answer of no fool.

October 5

Home, after nine weeks and two days. I sound like a schoolgirl crossing off the days. Everything as it was and as I wanted it to be. I seize on the hawthorne, loaded with scarlet berries (much nearer to scarlet at least than the hedge-thorns in England) as a symbol of the day.

I still want to write about the body and the soul and their debate in the old folks' home.

I woke and heard the Body and Soul talking.

Not in debate, orderly, as in the Middle Ages (when the Soul always won). I'd like to end with waking to the pagan sun all over the window and the thrust of a young tree in spring. Just now all the leaves are turning and quite beautifully when the light is on them.

October 6

My newest roommate, who is half-paralyzed and has to be lifted and who is generally very quiet and sweet-tempered, has just remarked—and not ill-temperedly—"I've got to get home. I'll walk bare-foot if I have to."

The voice of Theresa B. rises from across the hall, very deep, like a man's, "Nurse, I want to go to bed." They keep coming and telling her it's too early. What she wants, she wants. Her cry of "Nurse" is almost as loud as Frederick M.'s deaf bellow, which is intended to be the tone of conversation. "I had a beautiful bowel movement," he cries to the public at large.

Lucetta drenched me with a powerful scent when I paused to see her, as I always do on my walker. "I am blue. I cry all day. What can you do? I live-a too long but what you going to do?" Then she picks up her beads. "There is no one but our blessed Lord and the blessed Mother." When I leave she says, "God-a bless, Signora."

The Rev. Mr. M., after a nice conversation about language, worked me into his prayer and said, "We thank thee (he may have said *you*—they seem to nowadays) for the interpreters and we thank thee for this interpreter." I took this as a great compliment, though I know there's not much of the interpreter left in me. A consolation for what I heard one of the night nurses say, commenting on the patients to a new recruit. "She just gave up. She's 71 (inaccurate) and she's finished." (Afterwards I thought it may have been my roommate they were talking about, but she didn't give up.)

October 9

Listening to the St. Matthew Passion while I put cream on my face and felt at peace, in spite of the wet, grey day with the fallen leaves pressed into the wet road and the wretchedly inadequate light, no good for reading or writing. This is a beautiful recording from Blanche Moyse's lot—I wish I'd heard them once at Marlboro. Oddly enough the memories that keep piercing me are not of the St. Matthew at St. Bartholomew's, but the St. John and all my hearings of the St. John run together—"Ach mein Sinn" (?) at St. Bart's—the first time I'd every really listened to its intricacy, the woman weeping, and then the Tanglewood concert, when my feet got colder and colder but I wept over the "Ruhe Wohl" chorus, and then the very good performance at Mt. H. and the thrill of the opening chorus, the opening word. I suppose everything will run together more and more. . . . When I gave my roommate a brownie at supper last night, she said, "I'm keeping it for Mr. X." (her husband, who is dead), though in general her mind is clear.

October 15

Caught up in the politics of the place again (not the national campaign, though I did rouse myself this week to send J. Carter a *New York Times* editorial). Have spent the day, except for one beautiful hour outside, writing to doctors and politicians who might be interested in the survival of this place as it is, with a proper nursing service, therapy, etc.—a place where students can be brought for practice work and where no one is left to lie and rot, while some quite remarkable cures have been effected. It was interesting to find oneself at this age so activist.

Yesterday had my first poem of old age accepted—the "Words for Music" which I think my best of these late ones and which I like because it has in it the perfection of that Saturday we sat in the garden with Jo and the leaves had the movement of first snowflakes before the snow sets in in earnest, but the sun was warm on our backs and everything still but for the leaves.

October 20

Lucetta, my Italian Signora, has just come back from the hospital—she was taken there after a diabetic attack from which she soon recovered—and is crying as ever. She cries for sorrow and for joy. She cries that she is old and has had to leave home, that she ever left Italy (in 1913), that her son is married to a bad woman, but she blesses us all and prays to the Blessed Mother for us and I am glad to hear her voice again—one hears it rooms away—and shall welcome even her snores at night.

October 28

I don't think I'll ever finish or ever get a shape for the poem I want to write on the dialogue between the body and soul, because in a way it is my continuing dialogue that renews itself every day, but I did see an end—*"I was broad awake with the new day (sun?) at the window / and outside (beyond) an oak tree clinging to its leaves."*

A new man has just arrived in the ambulance for the room opposite, from which Peter C. has been evicted to the West Wing. I regret Peter C. as I regretted Mr. O. and Mr. H. He was the only conversible man in these parts. . . . Heard of the death of Martha Danielson, who used to call on so many people to help her, years ago it seems now. I'd like to think she was home.

Theresa next door crying "Nurse" in powerful tones that might well reach the nurses' station—unlike poor Florence's efforts next door on the other side (but Florence has been much quieter lately. I don't even hear her calling, "Bedpan, bedpan" in a morning). Theresa feels ill-used always, but that is partly because she is over 90, partly that she's deaf and half-blind. It is easy for the deaf to feel ill-used. Frederick M., the deafest of all, does not seem to—he does not act in an injured fashion—but he goes on reiterating his opinions or requests, almost expecting not to hear the other side. He is a big child, literally wanting to dress up for Halloween and excited about it.

November 1

He *did* dress up for Halloween, which achieved a kind of gaiety even, partly because some really young students who were here dressed up and danced with vigor and because Mrs. Maxwell —herself charming in her great-grandmother's brocade wedding dress and a big bonnet, had provided the therapy girls also with old clothes from her attic—how nice to think there are still people with trunks of family clothes in attics. Soon there will be neither trunks nor attics and the clothes saved will be in a museum.

The day was darkened, however, by the loss of Ellen, in many ways the ideal nurse, mother too and wife, I'm sure, and my political ally and my friend.

After being home, and with no connection, suddenly wrung with nostalgia for Maine in summer—the heart's intermittances —Proust knew about it young. Then ashamed that here I was indulging myself in this second-rate kind of emotion (I refuse to use the word *hedonic*) with someone in the room truly suffering and afflicted. And all mixed up with my feeling for Maine and Edna Clifford and the boys, a desire to write about them along with the flowers of lost Eden; then I said it all long ago and better than I could now.

November 7

This is Elizabeth's big day—in fact even now she may be making her speech in the chapel.

Someone at the other end of the wing is crying out "I'm dying. I'm dying," and again I feel how callous one becomes, in self-defense I suppose. I am calloused over most of the time with my roommate, but sometimes not. Last night, for instance, I was touched at her young son's conversation with her. (She is 70 but he is only 26.)* He is so big and strong and tries so hard—last night he was trying to get her to eat—to interest her, to get through to her. She talks perfectly rationally to him, and with a slight asperity at times which makes one feel she was full of no nonsense as a mother (she wanders only in time and in thinking her husband still alive). But there is pity in it, as if he would offer her anything, do anything to bring light into her face and too much is between them. The situation next door, with the little Polish woman, is worse, however, as her children do *all* the talking and she says nothing—there is really a wall between them. She *can* speak, as when they aren't there, she calls, "Nancy, Nancy, hurry up" and very occasionally, "Mark" and "Lillian." She sits in her chair, a tiny creature, as if there were only the shell of her there. No smile, ever, but neither does my roommate smile. Once a young nurse said to her, "Can't you smile?" and she said, "Not any more."

* Later I discovered he is 31.

November 8

The first snow—a flurry or not much more, a little on the ground and trees. It is too early! We are not ready. We are never ready for it.

November 10

Yesterday I passed a happy afternoon having a permanent wave, which would be incredible if it were not that I was with Elizabeth and Millie. I am so happy that Elizabeth was a real success and that everybody was delighted to have it so—or, if there were anyone who wasn't, I did not hear. I am happy it was one of the things with which nothing went wrong; the audience responded and R. Barrett afterwards told her what I'd told her before, that she knows more about Mary Lyon than anyone in the world. To-day—when we had much more of a snowfall but still not the real thing—I feel I am left among the ruins of whatever learning I had —I have been trying to talk Italian not to Lucetta but to Maria, who speaks an Italian I recognize, though I cannot wholly follow it. On top of that someone asked me about "No man is an island" and I was very fluent and professional but how little is left of what I once knew about Donne. Isn't there a poem—Auden?—about the ruined alphabets?

November 19

Again rejoicing with them that rejoice in that Anna Jane has been elected president of the American Chemical Society, the first woman. I don't know anyone fitter to receive honors, to be less puffed up by them, to carry them as if they didn't exist. She is the opposite of V.

Again caught up in local politics. After a series of indignation meetings over an editorial in the *Gazette*, which said Mr. Drake's proposal to change the rating of this place seemed a good one. I wrote to Irmina, thinking she might have a voice on the *Gazette* by this time—I know they think highly of her, but I was also in on some of the meetings—informal of course—in this room. They culminated in a clandestine meeting of some of the nurses—led by the invaluable Charles—down the road and off the county land, with a reporter from the *Gazette*. Now, today, it has just come over the radio that our employees want an explanation from the state and not from one man. It also said, "Their names are being withheld for fear of retaliation." For a moment we were embracing one another in high excitement. I felt as if I were in a small country trying to get its independence.

Yesterday, Mrs. Maxwell, introducing me to a visitor, called me a "stabilizing influence." I was never called that in my life before.

December 7

I am writing in the half-dark after a long silence (Christmas cards, which are still on top of me, stiff neck, lethargy, a feeling of grieving is more prolonged and intense than I've had before, partly for the want of companionship). Today it has been sleeting all day, after a night of it. On Saturday it snowed all day and I found myself—I was on my way somewhere else—in the West Wing, where the inhabitants were gathered in the sun parlor—no sun, but snow out of every window, very soft, not blowing. The trees like Christmas trees. And all the hopeless cases, the people with their mouths open, some asleep, the bright expectant face of Don R., who can't speak but looks out on the world, as if something were going to happen. And someone—a nurse's sister—playing carols on a little spinet electric piano, while the snow kept coming down, no expression—can one on a piano attached to batteries? —but the familiar airs, the quietness—very few had the power or sense to applaud—and yet it wasn't like "The Dead." There was a Peace on Earth feeling, though winter had come to stay—the snow looked as if it had settled on us perfectly. I wondered if it was because there is hope in carols, and a simplicity that clears the clutter of the world away for a moment—beginnings, a manger and shepherds and a star. But it is rather familiarity, something one has gone the whole way with, like Tobias's angel or at least his dog.

December 15

I should put down an afternoon of happiness, though the sky fell. It began with carol-singing—I want to go on singing them, only wish to sing more than one gets a chance to. I hummed to myself "Entre le boeuf" and "Masters in the Hall" as I walked in the corridor, after a visit from Elizabeth and Bea and the munificent gift from Elizabeth of *Country Life* and a beautiful (physically a beautiful piece of workmanship, with Maureen's printing and a friend's borders of small animals of the prairie) letter, life of Maureen and Peter since we last heard from them—and a letter from Joan in which she told me she was singing the *Laudamus Te* in the B Minor—had sung it, in fact, successfully though with a dry mouth. I feel like a grandmother (though how do I know?) over the successes of old students. Anyhow I want to cry and sing, whereas yesterday I was ready to lie down under the snow.

I ought to put down the old man who came in here in a wheelchair, his leg amputated, and asked if I knew where he could get a taxi. He had to get downtown, he said. And then there was the old woman in her wheelchair, trying to get out of the front door. I held her a moment, telling her they did not want her to go, till a nurse came and told her she must go back to her room. The woman said, "I haven't a room here (probably "don't have" is what she said). I've left." The nurse said, "Oh! come on, Esther. You live in the West Wing." Esther said, "It's ridiculous. I could get a job as a stenographer any time"—she in a housecoat and johnny, with her hair tied up on top with a ribbon. In her eighties?

When happiness comes to one so, in old age, it leaves one with the feeling that it may never come back. And it is not ecstasy. One is inside oneself, not beside. (Another thing I forgot about today was that it began, after the creature-comfort of my bath, with Beethoven's 3rd Piano Concerto, my favorite. And then went on to more Beethoven, including a sonata I like, remade as a quartet.) But it comes on one like other unexpected, unrepeated things— the bird seen once. I suppose I'm just saying all experience is unique and that in age any time may be the last time. Truisms.

December 23

There is so much I have intended to put down lately, but couldn't do it and write Christmas letters. Most of the letters were a pleasure—there were too many, that's all. But almost none of them perfunctory—a far cry from the hundreds sent out by important people with just a printed name. Changes happen so fast now, or I am so slowed down, that everything becomes much more like last week's news on the TV screen. We have had such processions of carollers, some good, some (e.g., a neighborhood group of little boys, cub scouts) pretty bad musically, but engaging. Some sixth graders from Easthampton brought us plaques covered with foil and a reindeer outlined on each one, effective in their way and bright on these bare walls. In the midst of all this I read May Sarton's *As We Are Now* about a nursing home which makes this seem heaven. I can't believe hers would have passed any kind of inspection, but I am not saying there are no such places, nor any such sadistic women as the proprietress. The thing that was interesting to me was the heroine (it seems the wrong word) and her notebooks, her loneliness and, in the end, madness. She discovered what I had discovered for myself—that nursing homes are purgatory. (I feel I should read the *Purgatorio* again), only I am on the lower slopes seeing the mountain rising above me but stopping there to listen to Casella. I felt I'd like to write to May Sarton and may yet.

Just now I am full of family feeling as well as old student feeling, having had letters not only from Susan, Elsie, and Thomas, but Ted—after a silence of I'd say forty years—Mildred, and "Cousin Bessie," then Gillian of the next generation. I count my blessings, with a feeling I ought to throw salt over my shoulder or curtsey to the moon or something.

Yet I feel also from time to time shame that I care less for the cries in the night, that I feel *dislike* of the man opposite, though he is very ill (Mrs. Maxwell says it is a wonder he is alive), when he bangs the sides of his bed at night and tears his bed apart and yells. I find him sinister looking and think very unreasonably, "Why can't he ring his bell?" when he's beyond it and can only struggle against his fetters and tear his clothes and shout. I am less ashamed of sometimes thinking Frederick M. an old fool, because he is so loudly happy in the midst of his egocentricity. (Yet he gets upset if any small thing goes wrong, e.g., if his paper does not arrive at the moment he expects it. He says, "Everything has to happen to me," though in another mood he glories in his wonderfulness at 89, a little like Mr. H. He says, "I believe I'm the best one in the lot.") Sometimes too, he is touching, as when he takes his hymnbook and sings carols tunelessly beside the blue, gauzy angels at the front door.

Charles, the tower-of-strength nurse who is going to the hospital after Christmas, has been telling Frederick M. he must walk when he's not there as when he is. And Frederick M. evades this by saying, "I'm so concerned about you, Charles." C., "I'm not talking about me. I want you to walk when I'm not here." F.M., "Yes, Charles, but I'm so sorry you've got to go through this." Ad infinitum. And F.M. *won't* walk when Charles is not there.*

December 29

A low day, yet not perhaps so low as yesterday. The sun is struggling out over the snow—two days' snow from a storm called Chris. I feel as if we've been paying ever since Christmas Day. Everyone seems fractious, except Grace who is never that. (She is just now asleep, with her hair, snow-white spread out on the pillow, with something about her head that reminds me of Greek friezes.) Ruth T. on the one side is making half-articulate cries and Ruth H. on the other, uttering her calling syllables half-sung which make her roommate (Florence, who cries like a child —it really sounds like *boo-hoo*, syllables I never believed when I saw them written) say, "Stop it." Theresa B. has come back after a month, I'd say, at the hospital. Her voice hasn't got the power back into it yet. I am sorry that the gentle, harmless but bewildered Mrs. L. has been moved, for her sake especially, as it will disorient her all over again. (It will also distress her nice roommate.) In another wing, she may even go back to wandering the corridor in her gloves, with her handbag, asking strangers where her room is. On the other hand I am glad to have lost the man who

---

* I turned out to be wrong about this.

shouted and banged—he's been moved farther up the wing. I don't know his medical history, but he had a fine-featured Machiavellian face with a thin mouth I could have been afraid of if we'd been at large. Actually I believe he was a rough farmer of no education and the politic monkish look was misleading. He yelled "Hey" and his response to the people who tied him up tended to be, "I'll have you in court for this."

But Christmas Day was wonderful, fine and sunny with the snow holding off till midnight. I went in the college limousine and the driver and I sang carols with the car radio all the fifteen miles home. Then there was the accustomed pleasure of packages opened by the fire, with the callers coming in at intervals, almost gay, with real food and wine and time to talk. I came back here at 8:30 with the glow still on me, the slump set in with the snow the next day and I'm still in it.

1977

January 4

The New Year itself worse than the post-Christmas slump because of the common cold which has hemmed me in since New Year's morning. For two days I felt I couldn't write thank yous for fear of betraying self-pity. Not even the fact that Jimmy Carter has invited me to the inauguration (i.e., invited me to a seat in the cold outside and the pleasure, if I wish it, of walking in the parade—with my walker?) could get me to the point of simulating liveliness.

Just now I feel like recording the wail of Theresa B. over the way (she is getting more power into her voice) that she does not want to be tied. She spaces her words carefully, sometimes accenting them as in French—bathróom. "Nurse, I don't want this brace. I don't need it. I never had such a thing before (false). Nurse, I don't want to be here. I want to be back where there are people I know." I wonder if she can envisage where she wants to be and how many people she knows are there? Not here anyway. She is in her nineties.

The other person who has been disturbing the afternoon, though not wailing, is Frederick M. He cannot grasp the fact that his roommate has had a stroke, that he is not incontinent from choice ("He's the filthiest fellow I ever saw") and perhaps stranger still that people have to lift his hands for him. "He doesn't shake hands like everybody else. They have to lift it up. It would be the same if it were the President of the United States." Then he goes and shouts this to someone else up the hall. "My bed's just as clean when I get up as when I go to bed. I don't have it changed but once a week. [The rule.] He has to have his changed every day. Of course I'm very careful." He reminds me of Mr. H. with poor old Mr. G.

January 9

Still nothing to be said for 1977. The last four days, this wing has been quarantined for the gastro-intestinal bug that is going up and down these vinyl halls. The first big snow lies thick on the ground with, just now, sun on it and some rather beautiful shadows which, however, fail to touch the heart. Tonight we are to have another. For a while, when it was coming down I listened, as last year, fascinated by the list of things cancelled—a new lot every half hour—and marveled at the number of clubs and organizations that had meetings and dances and Bingo games set for one January evening. I feel now that there will be one storm after another, that I'll never shake this cold, that I'll never get home, and that it will take a Paul Revere to get through to me.

January 12

Went to church in a fit of anger almost unprecedented here—first Mr. Drake's letter saying the prices were going up $9.00 a day as decided by the state, and then the sudden discovery that there was church and it was time for it and my chair had disappeared. I believe the state of mind is described as being ready to chew nails. I hardly listened to the service, only my eye caught the cheap color prints stuck on the wall in place of the Santa Clauses and reindeer and stars, a girl reading a letter, a girl looking out of a window—Vermeer perhaps or even Rembrandt among others—and I felt that is what life is, the piercing through a series of moments—only in age the stretches between are longer and longer. Even last year I did not feel I could not face winter as I do today. I took communion automatically. I could not even feel "Lord I am not worthy." When I thought about it afterwards, I couldn't be certain I wasn't being literary. It's hard to be honest when one's so damn literary. And I went back to thinking of Mr. Drake and his bald, unsigned notice and the horror of being a pauper so much sooner than I'd counted on. The darkness of the stretches between is our own darkness. No one but me can get me out of it. Bertile would say God could help; so would Ellen. Keith Thompson—who wrote to me the other day about my poem on the leaves falling, saying it described perfectly the feeling of transcendental meditation—would say I could pull myself out of it by T.M. Actually Mrs. Maxwell was wonderfully helpful and soothing to my ego and took half an hour of her own time to calm me down.

January 15

Last night for the first time I overcame my dislike and felt pity for Theresa B. It is the first time I've heard her without the edge of complaint and self-justification in her tone. She was saying over and over again, and quite quietly, "O seigneur, aidez-moi. Jésu, Marie, et Joseph, aidez-moi."

January 20

J. Carter inaugurated, not unimpressive in spite of the simplicity, because of it too, of his address. What I hope is that it has a simplicity that reduces the complications of the world. No eloquence, but no false eloquence either. The whole thing barely got through to me, however, as I was having one of the worst slough-of-despond periods I've had since I came here. I think conceivably a pill to reduce my heart-beat may have had something to do with it, as the last few days I've wanted to creep into my shell and stay there. Today nothing could rouse me, bands, horses, a letter asking me for suggestions for a memorial service for Griffy. I can think of loads of suggestions for my own memorial service, with self-pitying tears running down my cheeks.

Later heard Ruth H. next door, after one of the one-sided conversations with her son—though she talks a little more, sings or half-sings more—"I don't want to go nowhere." He had asked her, foolishly, I thought, "Do you want to come home with me or do you want to stay here?" Today I understood the feeling of not wanting to go anywhere except to sleep.

January 24

Well, Mrs. O. who was my roommate for six weeks or so has come back and already she has died. She went to that rest home in Easthampton jubilant because it was Easthampton, but did not last long there. She had been in the hospital nearly three months when they brought her back, a wreck of herself. I was fond of her, in spite of my feeling she wanted from me what I couldn't give. She was humble and small things were a treat to her. She could entertain herself endlessly with the catalogues I passed on to her. I could offer her very little, but the mass on my TV—she wasn't interested in the news. She still said, "I love you, Joyce," and I never said, "I love you too." I saw her bed wheeled out just now when I was in the hall. Death comes discreetly here—a bed wheeled out and then another wheeled in.

January 27

Curious effect of reading Elizabeth Drew on the campaign (over for good or ill) while an antiphonal plaint goes on between Theresa B. and her new roommate, who cries out against fate as much as herself. Perhaps they are better together—either would drive most people crazy. The new roommate, who is always calling for Elinor, is shriller, nearer to tears than Theresa. "Elinor, come and get me out. This is enough of this. I never did anything to you. Elinor, for God's sake." While Theresa keeps up her basso continuo, "I want my leather shoes. Bring me a cup of water. No one wants to help here. They are all stingy, stingy, stingy. Why don't *you* get me a glass of water?" "Elinor, we're all going crazy." "I want my shoes and my beads." For the moment I sit here as in the land of Goshen, but with terror at all the burdens, and guilt at not caring enough.

Walking, I passed Ronald Y., the monkish one, asleep in his chair. He was wearing a dark robe and still looked like a scheming cardinal in Roger Peyrefitte. A fine-featured face, very paintable.

194

Later I saw he had untied himself and was trying to put his "restraint" in with the dirty linen.

January 28

Theresa B. is now yelling "Come on, neighbor" over and over. Dotty is not the only one who had a bird's repetition. She has kept it up half an hour. Even her roommate whose word patterns are much more tangential is begging her to stop. What she wants is to be taken out of the geri-chair and the nurse has told her she must stay in it. "I'm just an old school-teacher," says the roommate, "but I'd untie you if I had help." Then she calls "Elinor." Oh! dear—there is nothing one can say or do. The roommate, Lorraine M., was in a wheelchair when I was walking and she said, hearing the powerful cries, "Do you suppose my house is on fire?" And I keep thinking, "Who is my neighbor?" Nobody in Bedlam. And yet there must be people who could get through to them.

February 1

There have been so many hours of the evening antiphonal between Theresa B. and Lorraine M., I can't begin to record it, except that last night it seemed to have reached a height—but who can say? At one point Theresa was saying over and over, "Help *me, me, me.*" In a way we are all saying that, but she has the most powerful voice. This morning she was quiet while Lorraine M. called alternately on Elinor, her daughter, and God to deliver her. And here we all are, in a "safe shelter" and warm while the icecap covers so much of the country and people freeze in their cars, and schools close, and factories close, and who can save us? I felt strange swathed in my hot packs, reading a horrific account of clouds of poison gas—one in Italy, one in Chicago—neither dealt with, all part of the struggle to have industry and save the economy and the natural world, which at the moment is holding everything paralyzed. Outside here it is beautiful—the blueness that goes with snow, bare trees and strong light without heat. The groundhog has undoubtedly seen his shadow. . . . All this to the accompaniment of *Morning Pro Musica,* with a fine program, ending with a live trio from Exeter School playing Beethoven and Mendelssohn in spirited fashion, the strings of life.

February 3

Slow and intolerable sloth. Theresa, calling "Nurse." This morning she was calling, "Bring me a spoon to eat my cereal." At about the fiftieth time someone went in and told her she'd already eaten it. There was something in the words and tone that made me think of the Big Bear. . . . Yesterday I essayed a little conversation with Lorraine M., who was looking for her room in a wheelchair. I told her which it was. She said out of a background of polite hospitality, "Won't you come in and rest yourself?" Last night her daughter actually appeared, a tall, personable young woman. But today it is as if she had never been.

I think nursing homes even twenty years from now, whatever they are like, will be less centered in the family than this. When I see the young nurses divorced (not only nurses of course) and think of children in day-care centers, I don't think there will be quite the same parent-child situation; neither the devoted children who visit nor the bitter parents who accuse their children of putting them here. They (the nursing homes twenty years from now) will also be less religious; that is, the patients will be less likely to have the habits and the trappings and the consolations of a religion. Sometimes I wonder how much consolation they get, when the mind has started wandering? Theresa B., for instance. And yet I suppose she'd be worse off without her beads. (When did the rosary come into use and was it part of the cult of Mary in the 11th? 12th? century. Is there anything Middle Eastern about the beads?) One night when she was praying aloud—"O Seigneur, venez, venez donc, aidez-moi, O Ste. Anne . . ." without pause and with increasing force as she added more holy names, until her voice seemed to swallow the sound of all the radios and TVs, I felt she had something of an O.T. prophet in her. She reminded me too of the cantor on our record of the Russian Orthodox church, in the part where his voice grows louder and louder and more peremptory. I feel a miserable weakling beside Theresa B.

196

February 14

One can't sing "Nu wilcom sumer," though it is a fine day for
this winter. Very low. Nothing to be said for age. Even the two
heart-shaped cookies that appeared on our lunch tray had too
much flour in them. Met Alan in the waiting room of the Cooley
Dickinson Hospital where I was sent for a blood test and found
him with two books on the Idea of Progress in his hands—he is
taking the course. What is more, he has just given three Winter
Term courses. I wanted to weep because I couldn't give a course
on anything at all, even age. *De Senectute*—what a lot of glossing
over of things, or so I remember it.

Other manifestations of Valentine's Day: an ice-cream cone,
pink, which I couldn't eat, but Elizabeth who had come over—the
sudden lift that one did not anticipate—managed to eat hers; a red
and white paper corsage which I am wearing; a touching Valentine from those faithful Easthampton school children who put in
so much time on us, including a charming portrait of the artist,
Sara La Liberté; a visit from Irene with her grandson (Mrs. R.'s
great-grandson) and a box of Valentine candy. I ought to be
ashamed of my inclination to pity myself. But I can't help wishing
I could eat. There was also Dr. Brewster's visit which had nothing
to do with St. Valentine and which angered me by his lack of interest in my symptoms. Well, maybe they are small beer.

My Machiavellian man died. He was 66.

February 16

Letter from Billie in which she speaks of the condition of her
son (37?), so covered with the nodules of skin cancer that he
can't lie on his back, or properly use his hands, and the process—
in the mind—of the changing of pain to something "perhaps
peaceful, at least not so overwhelmingly destructive." And Bertile
is in Texas, taking a friend for cancer treatment at a certain hospital in Houston because "someone had to." And our next door
neighbor is dying, while his wife, who has always been the invalid
—he built homes, climbed ladders, sowed seed—is rising to take
on her new part in a way that compels admiration. It seems one
spends half one's life in age being ashamed of oneself.

February 27

Rising to the surface again after a low period in which I could not eat or enjoy anything. Yesterday I was charmed by an article in *Country Life* on cats in church, with illustrations from medieval mss, an annunciation with a very real cat in it (impending evil, said the article) more attractive than the angel, and photographs of real church cats who had just come to live in certain churches and refused to go away. The sight of one on the verger's lap made me wish for a cat then and there. There was also a pleasant reference to a hermit in *The Golden Legend* (6th century) who had given up all his possessions for God's sake except his cat "with which he played oft and held it in his lap deliciously." That was exactly what the verger of St. Mary Riddifle was doing. (Article by Gareth M. Spriggs in Dec. 23, 1976.)

One sees here both the impatience and the patience of the old, more of the first. Nothing could be more patient than my roommate, who has to be lifted, often with pain. But there is far more of the Theresa kind of thing. "Nurse, get my beads—get my beads (repeated several times). Nurse get me my garters. I *want* them now." . . . Meanwhile oil tankers sink or run aground, oil spills by the thousands of gallons, the West is devoured by drought and Idi Amin holds up American missionaries.

Automatically, turning the calendar, I think of Dorothy Wordsworth putting on her woodland dress and William and Dorothy giving this one day to idleness. All mine are given to idleness.

The Rev. Matthew has come back amongst us and has been put in a room with Frederick M., who has no idea and probably never will have of Mr. Edwards' mental state. It is just as well he can't hear him talking—perhaps that is why they put them together. But this morning F.M. was praying aloud, first extempore, thanking God for his blessings, then going on to the Lord's Prayer, in which the Rev. Matthew joined. This was at breakfast. After that the Rev. yelled his name and counted up to ten several times and F.M. tried to tell him how nice it was to go to crafts. It was like Beckett—except that the atmosphere is not that of the vacant lot and the ash can and F.M. at least is happy.

March 3

Today F.M. explained to the Rev. Matthew that he liked to take his hymnal to Bingo and sing a few hymns while he was waiting for the game to begin. He then got out the book and sang some then and there: "Abide with me," "Nearer my God to thee," the Rev. Matthew occasionally joining in. F.M. sings with no idea of pitch whatsoever and the result is dreadful and touching. After that the Rev. kept up a stream of inconsequence, including bits of hymns—he has developed the trick of sticking on the phrase, like a worn-out record—and once to my surprise "I warmed both hands before the fire of life / It sinks and I am ready to depart." He is now keeping on in the religious vein, so markedly absent from his conversation last time he was here. Whether it is F.M. that has opened it, or whether he had got down to his professional stratum in his sojourn in the South Wing, I've no idea.

I also have been preoccupied with hymns, since Muriel's gift —to be her last, she says—of the Methodist Hymnal. It had given me great pleasure to pick out tunes I'd forgotten and to discover that the Meth. Hymnal now includes "St. Patrick's Breastplate" and "God be in my head," which we sang at St. Hilda's on our knees, and several things like "Ein Feste Burg" which I was introduced to in the Guiseley School hymnal. "St. Patrick's Breastplate" I first encountered at Leeds Girls High School. Hymn-singing was part of my life till the end of college. There was one hymn, "I think when I read that sweet story of old," which I think of as a cricketing hymn, when I went with my father in the wagonette to wherever Robin Hood was playing "away"—once, I remember, to Barwick-in-Elmet: the long summer day in the open air, usually with Dorothy and Stanley Giles, with very little watching of cricket, but the pleasant atmosphere of a cricket-field in good weather, and the ride home, after high tea, with the men singing gospel hymns in harmony—what I think of as pub harmony, though I've never actually heard singing in a pub. "Beauteous scenes on earth appear" was a favorite. Going with the cricketers was one of my ideas of bliss before the age of ten.

March 4

By a coincidence we had, for the first time, a hymn singing at the church service. Mrs. Henderson had gathered up a few patients and a few employees of the hospital who could sing and the whole congregation had a wonderful time, not wanting to stop, though Mr. Montgomery, understandably, was getting restive, wanting to get on to *his* part of the service, which was communion.

March 9

Life increasingly made up of bits and pieces, fleeting memories arriving suddenly from nowhere, all the different stages of one's life offering a moment's glimpse—an attitude held, a sensation of weather, words out of context. I fasten on new facts in the same patchwork fashion. I was delighted to discover, for instance, that Gray's "little chaos" near his fox-hunting uncle's was Burnham Beeches and that J. Austen got her idea for Sotherton from a visit to Stoneleigh Abbey—also to learn for the first time the use of *terrier* for a land map in Trollope and suddenly to realize why a terrier dog is so-called.

March 22

It doesn't seem possible I should have let so much time go, especially as I've spent hours in sheer idleness, not very Wordsworthian. I see a future in which I shall do nothing, think nothing, see nothing. But that would be preferable to Lorraine M.'s constant anxiety (I hope she is not anxious in dreams) to find her mother, her father, her room, which every time one points out to her, she refuses to recognize. She says at times, "I think I'll take another apartment," at times, "I'm not staying here." There is an element of Beckett in her conversations with Theresa B., too. Both are inconsequent, though T.B. has her relatively lucid moments (also silent ones) and L.M. has none and L.M. *has* to speak—wail —while T.B. speaks loud and clear only when she wants anything or does not want whatever it is they are doing to her. One night, when T.B. was calling for Bertha (her granddaughter) and L.M.

joined in and called Bertha too, T.B. said, "Shut up, you don't know my relations." Once she said, "Shut up, *please.*" L.M. is so anxious to help too, though her favorite cry, after "Elinor" and "Mary," is "Help me." One day when T.B. was yelling for a bedpan, L.M. in her high soprano started calling, "Elinor, bring a bedpan for the lady," which after a number of repetitions turned into "Bring a bedpan for Elinor." Meanwhile Elinor comes every day and wheels her about, very kind and competent and well dressed. (L.M. has nice clothes too.) While E. is here, L.M. is quiet —and in her sleep, one supposes.

My other Beckett conversation, the one between Frederick M. and the Rev. Matthew, is ended forever. F.M. dropped dead on March 10. As everyone says, a good way to go. He was happy here and had no pain and could be completely absorbed in making large cocks of seeds and dried peas and other oddments in the craft class. He was 89 and had just about run out of money— hence *felix opportunitate.* I'd like to die so, but before 89. As for the Rev. Matthew, they've moved him again. I can't regret it. He was too much of a reminder. His language was breaking down, though not his volubility. He was "ugly" to the female nurses, calling them devils and saying once, "Oh! Lord, sweep them into hell," like the chaff in that bloody-minded harvest hymn.

March 28

Yesterday, when someone opened the door, a cat came in, not one of the wild ones who live outside but someone's pet who had strayed. It was a flower of a cat, all the things I like, pansy-tiger markings and a round face and big paws. It stirred all the ailurophile in me as I was allowed to pet it a few moments, to loud purrings and beautiful cat gestures. I thought of the hermit who gave up all but his cat.

My watch is running down, along with my knees. I can buy a new watch and shall have to. At the same time I hanker after a new dress, which seems folly. What is that Hardy poem, "When I behold my face / And view my wrinkled skin" and at the moment my downtrodden-looking hair. Yet I still want a new dress. Renouncing the world is hard.

Poor L.M. distressed this morning because they wouldn't let

her telephone her mother in the grave. She knew the number to call too.

Today for the first time I felt my legs were not going to make it back to my room. Today also my watch finally stopped.

April 15

Strange how the heart is suddenly wrenched after a period when it seemed shut as an oyster. I was looking at a card of Rottingdean in a high sea and remembering how Susan and I used to fight our way round the curve from Brighton to Rottingdean against wind and weather. Then I remembered Mother and her "Fireside Competition" in which she had to "solve" half a dozen pictorial representations of places each week and bought a post office guide, which we read at times with mirth, as over "Pratt's Bottom." I remembered Mother coming on *Rottingdean* and raising the very good question, "How would you *draw* Rottingdean?" I saw someone with gaiters devoured by worms. I suppose these visitations after another's death are no newer or stronger than the ones of absent people in life. One feels as if beams have crossed, but they haven't. I always go through the same useless regrets afterwards, that I was so full of myself even when I was old enough to know there wasn't too much there. It might have been excusable in the season of budding and promise. I once wrote a sonnet—lost—about getting impatient with Mother's slow pace when I wanted to fly "on the moulting wings of middle age." It's one of the ones I lost.

April 17

The visit of William Meredith yesterday gave me a slight lift or at least a change of position. I thought perhaps I might send out a poem or two. It was extraordinarily nice of him to penetrate here because he had seen me at all the other Glascock Poetry Contests when he'd been a judge.

T.B. woke me this morning and made me laugh—at 7 A.M.— by yelling, "Open the bar." I take it she wanted the side of the bed down. Sometimes she strays into a gallicism as today, later, when she yelled, "Nurse, I want to go to the cabinet," and often she leaves off *s* with a plural: "The nurse don't come because they don't want to come." But sometimes she has something neither French nor English like "Open the light."

May 17

If ever I am going to write in this book again it should be today because it is the perfection of a summer day, 90° but with a strong, almost a seaside wind. I sat down under the trees with M.C. and admired the bluets in the grass and something I can't put a name to, round the bases of the trees—white, with a lily-of-the-valley-like leaf and flowers more spikey than lilies, with long stamens, very pretty. I heard an oriole. Felt as if I were gulping in life in mouthfuls.

A very nice visit from Alfred on Saturday, utterly unexpected. He brought a newspaper picture of Hetsy, himself, and John, three Avery Hopwood prizewinners. Hetsy looking as proud as punch. Alfred makes one feel more alive, almost as if one could write. It is as if he believed everyone could write. Anyhow he cheered me up. What luck to have had Hetsy as an honors student, and to think I'm writing to another honors student's daughter and that this winter I had a letter on my *Commonweal* poem from my first honors student's son.

L.M. this morning, after calling on Elinor and Mary, began calling on Jesus to help. She wanted a bedpan, which with a half reversion to childhood she called a "potty-pan." She said, "Jesus, get them to bring me a potty-pan." But in childhood one made very small bargains with God—all one's immediate wants if they were strong enough. She often says, "I'll do anything for you." I don't know that she made any bargain with him this morning, but she did at one point say, "Hurry up, Jesus." Later she dropped several notches and began calling, "Operator." Later still, when she was up and dressed, she began to worry—out loud, of course —because her bed looked as if someone had slept in it. The nurse could not convince her that it was she herself.

Reading about Bernard Leach's pots in C. *Life,* I was struck by his having said, as the reason why there was a dying out of peasant art, "*We inherit everything* and we stand alone." (Italics mine.) That is why the TV news every now and then gets one down or one recoils from it. Everything is too much.

May 26

A perfect day, though one needed the sun. Wind and a mackerel sky, full of reminders of Maine and of a picture (artist unknown) I once pinned up on my wall in Frederick, of two Victorian ladies in windblown skirts looking up at such a sky of blue and white, it was called "The Lark"—and made me wish I could hear a lark again, still more see one going up all the way as we did that day on Dartmoor.

Today I committed myself to have the knee operation if they think fit.

June 13

Sunday was one of the worst days I ever put in here. I went to sleep in the afternoon out of pure boredom and I used to say I was never bored. La Rochefoucauld was right, "We can forgive those who bore us but we cannot forgive those whom we bore," and that works for ourselves. I bored myself, wanting to read nothing, having nothing to write. The day was grey, with rain threatening. If the sun had been out and I could have sat on the back-door step, just staring into the woods at birches and maples and fern and mountain laurel, the whole day would have changed. But even that wouldn't have given me my zest back again. Perhaps I've run through myself as well as the place.

I am tired of chronicling the wails of L.M. which go on and on but I must put down one thing she said, among other petitions, "Jesus, bring me my mother—and a cup of tea." I thought if I could see my mother, I'd want a cup of tea. So would she, though she'd be horrified with a tea bag in a styrofoam cup.

Today I was cheered by a letter from Alfred who is actually typing my journal—I can't get over such generosity—and as usual he raised my spirits and made me feel "I'm not dead yet." He said among other things that it did not make him feel *he* was in a nursing home, only that I was. And I suppose that is because it's a journal and hit or miss. There is so much of the ambience I take for granted. For instance I could go and find out what the society of the solarium is really like. If I were writing a novel I'd have to. Or I could put down what happened in a single day, beginning with the rushed getting up, the hard toast at breakfast and going on to washing and hot packs, but I can't imagine for whom.

June 27

Well, the die is cast as far as going to Boston is concerned, but the stakes are unknown. It may be that they will send me home after examining me, or *evaluating* as they say now, or it may be I am in for worse pain than I've ever had. I go blindly in the South Hadley ambulance.

Now that I am leaving the place, though maybe not for long, I realize how wedded I am to the routine which becomes almost pleasant. What I'll miss most in the way of physical comforts are the chair, first and foremost—not to be able to press a button and get up myself—and the tub baths, with the weekly delicious lowering into hot water and the feel of being able to splash instead of just keeping oneself clean from a basin and in a chair. And of course I'll miss the woods and the smell of grass new-mown and the smell of pine.

Library of Congress Cataloging in Publication Data
Horner, Joyce Mary, 1903–
That time of year.
  1. Horner, Joyce Mary, 1903–   —Diaries.
  2. Horner, Joyce Mary, 1903–   —Biography—Last years
and death. 3. Nursing homes—Massachusetts.
  4. Authors, English—20th century—Biography. I. Title.
PR6015.0685Z476   1982   828'.91203   [B]   81–23128
ISBN 0–87023–367–X   AACR2